ADVANCE

Nine Months Strong

"Bridson does a fabulous job of demystifying fitness during pregnancy and helping pregnant women prepare both physically and emotionally for their own marathons of labor."
—LISA STONE, Founder and President, Fit For 2, Inc., Pre- and Post-Natal Fitness Program

"Written in a practical and engaging tone, *Nine Months Strong* provides answers to a myriad of questions about getting in shape for pregnancy, birth, and postpartum. In this clear and concise roadmap for a healthy, fit pregnancy, Bridson proves that the ideal birth is not a stroke of luck but requires knowledge, effort, and dedication. An outstanding guide—required reading for anyone planning on having a baby."
—JULIA ROSIEN, Senior Editor, ePregnancy.com

"A testimony to the rewards of training for the marathon of pregnancy and beyond. Ms. Bridson takes the reader step by step through the training of this sport we call pregnancy—what to expect, how to prepare, what to do, how to succeed, and how to go beyond the finish line. Bravo to Ms. Bridson and *Nine Months Strong*!"
—BESS HILPERT, President, Mothers In Motion, Inc.

"Women already know how to run everything from marathons to corporations. This well-written book shows how they can apply those same goal-setting and motivational skills to preparing for childbirth."
—LINDA WASMER ANDREWS, author of *Scientific American Focus: Of Mind and Body*

Nine Months Strong

Nine Months Strong

SHAPING UP FOR LABOR AND DELIVERY AND THE TOUGHEST PHYSICAL DAY OF YOUR LIFE

KAREN BRIDSON

WITH KARIN J. BLAKEMORE, M.D., MEDICAL ADVISOR

LifeLine Press

A Regnery Publishing Company, Washington, D.C.

Copyright © 2004 by Karen Bridson-Boyczuk

All rights reserved. No part of this publication may be reproduced or transmitted in any form or by any means electronic or mechanical, including photocopy, recording, or any information storage and retrieval system now known or to be invented, without permission in writing from the publisher, except by a reviewer who wishes to quote brief passages in connection with a review written for inclusion in a magazine, newspaper, or broadcast.

Original illustrations by Patrisha Tamariz, with the exception of medical illustrations on pp. 46–47: copyright Johns Hopkins University, Department of Art as Applied to Medicine.

Library of Congress Cataloging-in-Publication Data

Bridson, Karen.
  Nine months strong : shaping up for labor and delivery and the toughest physical day of your life / Karen Bridson-Boyczuk with medical advisor, Karin Blakemore.
    p. cm.
  Includes bibliographical references and index.
  ISBN 0-89526-091-3
  1. Labor (Obstetrics) 2. Delivery (Obstetrics) 3. Pregnancy. I. Blakemore, Karin. II. Title.
  RG651.B756 2004
  618.4--dc22
                    2004001637

ISBN 0-89526-091-3

Published in the United States by
LifeLine Press
A Regnery Publishing Company
One Massachusetts Avenue, N.W.
Washington, DC 20001

Visit us at www.lifelinepress.com

Distributed to the trade by
National Book Network
4720-A Boston Way
Lanham, MD 20706

Printed on acid-free paper
Manufactured in the United States of America

10 9 8 7 6 5 4 3 2 1

Books are available in quantity for promotional or premium use. Write to Director of Special Sales, Regnery Publishing, Inc., One Massachusetts Avenue, N.W., Washington, DC 20001, for information on discounts and terms or call (202) 216-0600.

The information contained in this book is not a substitute for medical counseling and care. All matters pertaining to your physical health should be supervised by a health care professional.

*For my son, Adlai,
the best run partner a woman could hope for
(both in utero and in baby jogger!),
and for my mother, Judi,
who didn't teach me how to run,
but taught me how to fly.*

Contents

Acknowledgments ix
Preface xi
Why Train Your Body for Labor and Delivery? xv

| 1 | Pregnancy Fitness Basics 1
| 2 | Building Cardio Fitness 19
| 3 | Getting Strong 41
| 4 | Open Up with Yoga 81
| 5 | Preparing Your Vagina and Breasts for Baby 105
| 6 | Eating for Two 119
| 7 | Getting Mentally Fit for Baby 147
| 8 | The Power of Rest 165
| 9 | Countdown to the Big Day 177
| 10 | The Big Day 183
| 11 | Positions for Labor and Delivery 197
| 12 | Natural Supports 207
| 13 | Backups You May Need 217
| 14 | Recovery 223
| 15 | Getting Back in the Game 233

Acknowledgments

I would first like to thank Dr. James Clapp III for his groundbreaking research into pregnancy fitness, which has not only been the foundation for this book and many others, but has given active women the freedom and reassurance needed to keep doing what they love. I would also like to thank Dr. Clapp for his feedback during the research for this book. Thanks also to Dr. Elizabeth Joy and Dr. Jane Katz for their invaluable expertise and feedback. And special thanks to yoga instructor Shasta Townsend from the Balanced Life Yoga Studio in Uxbridge, Canada for her direction and expertise. For their expertise and guidance, thanks to Pilates expert Phyllis Douglas, prenatal yoga expert Amy Berry, physiotherapist Shelle Jones, doula Sasha Padron, and midwife Carla Stange. Thanks also to the Melpomene Institute and Judy Mahle Lutter for their trailblazing study and research in women's sport and fitness. Thanks also to the many women who shared their stories of exercising in pregnancy with me. I must also thank my editor at LifeLine Press, Molly Mullen Ward, whose faith, passion, and vision got this book off the ground. Thanks to Beth Mottar and the rest of the LifeLine team. Thanks also to my husband, Bob, who heard me ranting one day about how I was going to train for my delivery the way I trained for my marathons and suggested it would make a great book. Thanks also to my father, Jim, the former high school track star, who gets so proud when he sees me run across the finish line. And a very special thank you goes to Karin J. Blakemore, M.D., without whom this book could not have happened. Her expertise, knowledge, and feedback were invaluable during the writing of this book. Finally, thank you to my mother, Judi, for carrying me for nine months, putting up with me for thirty years, and loving me always.

Preface

So you're pregnant! You're thrilled. It's all you can think about. That precious little bundle of joy is so quickly growing in your belly. It's natural to want to sit around in cute maternity wear, making plans and dreaming about the day you can hold your sweet child. And this is exactly what you should be doing; at least, that is, some of the time. But we can't forget that having a baby is hard work, and I mean that starting *now*. We all know caring for a newborn ranks among the most difficult jobs on the planet, but in the foggy delight of early pregnancy, too few of us realize just how hard the pregnancy itself, the labor and delivery, and early motherhood will be on our bodies as well as our minds. More critically, too few of us realize that we can—and should—be working to ready ourselves physically and mentally for those challenges that have already begun.

    This realization came to me about halfway through my pregnancy. I began to worry a great deal about the pain of my upcoming labor. I had heard gruesome tales of agony, and I worried that I wouldn't be able to cope. I wanted to avoid using medical interventions, like an epidural (an injection in the spine to numb all pain), if possible, but I feared I wouldn't be able to manage without it. That's when the idea struck me that I should approach this pregnancy and delivery the way I had approached the three marathons I had run: I would treat the upcoming Big Day just like any other highly intense physical challenge. I would train, I would plan, I would visualize the event, I would carbo-load, I would do everything I would do in preparation for running a marathon.

And boy was I glad I did. Giving birth and the postpartum period were the hardest physical challenges of my life. The marathons I have run don't even compare. In fact, when I "hit the wall" running my fourth marathon seven months after the birth of my son and found myself staggering to the finish line, I remember thinking, "This still isn't as bad as labor!"

So, although it may be tempting much of the time during your pregnancy, sitting around eating bonbons while picking out baby clothes isn't going to make the hard physical work of pregnancy any easier. In fact, doing that will make it all harder on you physically. Keeping your body strong as it works to accommodate your pregnancy is critical to a healthy and comfortable pregnancy, an easier and faster delivery, and a quick, enjoyable recovery.

Training Defined

Whether you simply want to continue to be active through your pregnancy or strengthen your body for the first time during pregnancy, this book will help you to arrive at labor day feeling strong. Designed like an actual marathon training guide, it will walk you through every step of preparing your body and mind for the different stages of pregnancy, labor and delivery, and the immediate postpartum period. Chapters will focus on such things as improving your cardiovascular endurance, strength, and flexibility and preparing your vagina and breasts for birth and baby. We will look at what to eat and drink in pregnancy, in the days leading up to delivery, and during labor; how to prepare your mind for labor and early motherhood; and what physical positions can help ease the pain of labor and speed delivery. We'll also focus on the importance of rest, counting down to the Big Day, specific details of the delivery itself, and how to have a quick recovery. You'll learn the art of squatting, how to prepare your upper and lower back for carrying baby (pre- and postnatally), how to strengthen the abdominal muscles used in labor, how to stretch your perineum (vagina) in preparation for delivery, how to toughen and shape your nipples for breastfeeding, how to breathe effectively, how to calm your mind, and much more. Ultimately you will strengthen the muscles needed from head to toe to feel strong in labor and early motherhood.

What You'll Be Doing

The most important first step in any prenatal fitness program is to have a thorough medical exam and discuss your exercise plans with your health practitioner. While a woman having a healthy, uncomplicated pregnancy can usually continue with most fitness regimens, there are a number of medical situations in pregnancy that can make certain forms and levels of exercise dangerous. So be sure to check with your health practitioner before proceeding.

The first section of this book focuses on the physical exercise component of preparing for baby. Cardiovascular fitness, strength training, and flexibility are three key elements of any fitness program. While it's important that the program you set out for yourself encompass elements from each of these areas, you don't have to do every exercise in this book. What you need to be doing is some kind of cardiovascular workout three to four times a week, strength-training exercises for all the major muscle groups one to two times a week, and muscle stretches before and after each of these workouts. (Note: If you have not been active prior to pregnancy, you must wait until the second trimester to start any significant exercise program other than walking. See page 22 for the first-trimester walking program for new exercisers.)

Chapter Two, Cardio Fitness, gives you the choice of four modes of exercise: two weight-bearing (walking and running) and two non-weight-bearing (cycling and swimming). It's up to you which you feel most suits your lifestyle and preferences. You can also do some of each, making sure to have a total of at least three cardio workouts each week. Throughout the book, however, there will also be a number of highlighted exercises targeting specific areas that need strengthening or specific work. In many of these cases, it's recommended you do these exercises every day, and in some cases, several times a day.

Now, let's take a closer look at just why it is you would want to train your body for pregnancy, labor, and motherhood.

Why Train Your Body for Labor and Delivery?

The changes brought on by pregnancy can boggle the mind. Your internal organs get relegated to remote locales, your feet disappear beneath your ever-growing belly, your ankles, face, and hands become nearly unrecognizable, your body is plagued by a whole host of new ailments, and the bathroom scale starts coming up with numbers you've never even seen before. And this is just the tip of the iceberg.

While most of these changes are well outside of our control—and *should* be for the health of the baby and ourselves—there are a number of things we can do to help our bodies adjust to these new demands and prepare for the challenges that lie ahead.

Physical Health Benefits for You

The physical health benefits of exercising through your pregnancy are extensive. Exercise limits weight gain and fat retention; improves cardiovascular function and endurance; lessens nausea, fatigue, backache, and many other pregnancy ailments; and can actually leave you in better cardiovascular condition than you were in before you became pregnant.

During my own pregnancy, I went for regular runs up until three days before I went into labor. While my distance and speed greatly diminished as my belly grew bigger, those runs were critical to keeping my body and mind healthy and strong while getting me ready for labor. My runs also helped alleviate the swelling, headaches, and backaches the pregnancy caused. In addition to running, I practiced yoga throughout my pregnancy, focusing on various stretches and strengthening exercises like pelvic tilts and squats. These exercises, and the Kegels and manual perineum stretching I did, were all key in helping me through my labor. As a result, my delivery nurse commented on how much control I had over my abs and pelvic floor during the pushing phase of labor. As for perineal tearing (tearing in the area between the vagina and the anus), I suffered the lowest grade of perineal tearing possible (short of none at all!) during my son's delivery.

While all of these measures were critical to my surviving the first seventeen hours of my labor, ultimately I had an epidural. This was something I was hoping to avoid, but I am sure that I never would have made it that far drug-free (I had another four hours to go) had I not prepared the way I did. And, had my labor progressed more quickly, I believe I could have made it through without drugs.

My delivery experience and subsequent life with my son made me hungry to learn more about how I could have done an even better job of preparing my body for this powerful transformation. This book is a compilation of all the current expertise in this area. Whether you hope to go drug-free or opt for varying levels of medical intervention for your comfort, there are plenty of things you can do in the months leading up to labor and delivery that can make your mind and body more prepared.

For instance, through certain exercises, you can lessen the backaches that torment most pregnant women. As our babies and bellies grow, our pelvis tilts forward, causing our lower back muscles to work harder, become shortened, and tighten up. Consequently, the opposing muscles in our abdomen stretch and lose strength and tone. This ultimately leads to lower backache during and after pregnancy and can diminish our power to push the baby out in the delivery room. There are a number of exercises we can do to strengthen these overburdened muscles and help counter these effects.

Also, the postural changes that accompany pregnancy cause our upper backs to round out, our shoulders to internally rotate and slump, and our heads to jut forward. At the same time, the growth of our breasts and caring for a child put new demands on these already stretched-out and weakened upper back muscles. Left unconditioned, these muscles can be another source of painful backaches in pregnancy and early motherhood.

By strengthening our leg muscles, we create a strong foundation for our bodies during labor and delivery and those long nights walking the halls with baby. Lower body exercise can also prevent varicose veins in pregnancy.

Gaining overall endurance with cardiovascular workouts will improve our overall fitness and limit weight gain while helping provide the stamina needed in labor and early motherhood.

Our arms are another area of our bodies that need particular attention heading into motherhood. While strong arms are needed to assist in positioning yourself for comfort during labor, they are essential to holding your child after birth without the overuse injuries commonly associated with new parenthood.

We can also prepare ourselves for delivery with Kegel exercises, manual perineum stretching, and yoga. Kegels teach us how to relax our pelvic floor muscles for the pushing stage of labor while helping to prevent urinary incontinence, a common side effect of vaginal birth and pregnancy. Yoga and flexibility training can also help us to "open up" our pelvis, learn to relax, and take control of our breathing—all important elements of delivery preparation.

Weight Management

Despite all of these benefits, the most well known and sought-after benefit of exercising in pregnancy is probably combating excessive weight gain. Many pregnant women start thinking about exercise sometime around the second trimester, when their waists disappear, their arms start to thicken, and their bums widen due to rising hormone levels and the increasing size of the baby. Many worry that if they allow weight gain to get out of control early in pregnancy, the amount they will ultimately have to lose may become unmanageable.

On average, North American women gain between fifteen and sixty pounds during their pregnancies, with twenty-five to forty pounds being the recommended weight-gain range. Studies done by leading pregnancy exercise researcher Dr. James Clapp III, author of *Exercising Through Your Pregnancy*, found that one year after delivery, the average weight retention of nonexercisers was three times greater and the fat retention was two times greater than those of exercisers.

Gaining excess weight can lead to a number of ailments during pregnancy, including backache and gestational diabetes (a high blood sugar condition in pregnancy that can cause serious problems for mother and baby). In fact, the American Diabetes Association has endorsed exercise as "a helpful adjunctive therapy" for gestational diabetes. Exercising in pregnancy can also lower the risk of preeclampsia (a potentially harmful condition marked by high blood pressure that can lead to premature delivery), with activities like jogging, stair-climbing, swimming, and cycling giving the greatest benefits. For these reasons and many more, keeping your gains within the recommended norms is extremely important for all pregnant women, and exercise is the best way to safely do that.

"Women should be encouraged to exercise in pregnancy," says Dr. Elizabeth Joy, sports medicine doctor and Associate Professor of Family and Preventative Medicine at the University of Utah. "Exercise is something that can prevent many problems.... This is huge for mother and baby." Dr. Joy adds that her fit patients don't tend to get stretch marks—a benefit of exercise that might be all the motivation many moms-to-be need to take on a pregnancy fitness program. Regular exercise also increases the amount of energy you can generate, the amount of oxygen you can use, and the amount of fat you can burn even during times of rest. Also, regular exercisers experience a reduction in their body's stress response to exercise, making it easier for them to cope with all kinds of physical challenges, such as an unexpected climb up five flights of stairs when an elevator is on the fritz. Ultimately, keeping healthy throughout your pregnancy will make you feel strong come labor day and help you bounce back to your fitter former self more quickly.

Emotional Health Benefits

One of the biggest benefits of exercising through your pregnancy is the remarkable impact fitness can have on your emotional state. One in five pregnant women suffers from depression in pregnancy, according to a University of Michigan study published in the *Journal of Women's Health* in May 2003. Due to the overwhelming physical and emotional changes of impending motherhood, pregnant women can also suffer from body-image and self-esteem problems, poor outlooks, and anxiety. Not only can this make your pregnancy less enjoyable than it should be, but severe emotional difficulties may have a negative effect on the baby. On the other hand, women who exercise during pregnancy report better attitudes and mental states than their sedentary counterparts, maintaining a positive attitude about themselves, their pregnancy, and the upcoming labor and birth. In fact, a study conducted at the University of Melbourne in 2000 on the body image and psychological well-being of pregnant women showed exercisers had a reduced frequency of anxiety and insomnia, a higher level of psychological well-being, and a better body image.

Labor and Delivery Benefits

Ask any labor and delivery nurse and she'll tell you her more active patients tend to have shorter, easier, and less complicated labors. While the official jury is still out on whether exercising can truly have this kind of impact on labor and delivery, the evidence is mounting in support of this belief. Some of the most compelling evidence comes from Dr. Clapp's studies, which have found women who have participated in regular weight-bearing exercise throughout their pregnancy have labors that are one-third shorter than those of their sedentary counterparts. His studies also found:

- 35 percent decrease in the need for pain relief
- 75 percent decrease in the incidence of maternal exhaustion
- 50 percent decrease in the need to rupture membranes
- 50 percent decrease in the need to induce or intervene due to abnormal heart rate
- 55 percent decrease in the need for episiotomies
- 75 percent decrease in the need for surgical intervention

Other studies have reported that women who stay fit during pregnancy have elevated levels of b-endorphin during labor and delivery, which is believed to reduce their pain perception. Meanwhile, still others say exercise can't shorten or lessen the pain of labor but can help women "frame their pain." In other words, they believe that women who have put themselves through physical challenges in the past have a point of reference and more enlightened perspective when it comes to labor.

Also, while some researchers dispute the belief that exercisers have fewer cesareans or use fewer drugs during delivery, many doctors report anecdotal evidence of active women having easier deliveries. All agree, however, that being physically fit will help you deal with the stress of labor and delivery both physically and mentally, help you to relax in the first stage of labor and push in the second stage of labor, and give you more endurance. Ultimately, women who are able to exercise throughout their pregnancies also have better energy levels after their babies are born, which is much needed when you feel like you've been hit by a Mack truck—as so many new moms do!

How Exercise Helps Your Baby

Much of the controversy over working out during pregnancy, I believe, is tied to the idea that women are bad mothers if they ever put themselves first. While this is not true in any case, know this: You are not putting your own goals for physical and emotional well-being ahead of your child's health when you decide to exercise during pregnancy. In fact, exercise is good for your baby in many ways. First, the motion of aerobic activity can be soothing for the baby. My son slept through every run I went on in my pregnancy. Also, the hormones released during exercise pass across the placenta, and the baby gets a lift from your epinephrine. In early pregnancy, moderate exercise improves the growth of the baby and the growth of the placenta. Science has also shown mother's exercise during gestation decreases the amount of fat on the baby and improves stress tolerance.

All aspects of growth and development after birth in babies of exercising moms are equal to or better than those observed in nonexercising moms, studies have shown. In fact, Dr. Clapp's investigations found the one-year-olds of exercising moms do better on standardized intelligence tests. At five years old, these children show no physical difference, but the exercising moms' children score much higher on general intelligence and oral language skills. While I suspect these last findings may be more a result of the genetic makeup of the women who choose to continue exercising through pregnancy, these outcomes provide evidence that women can exercise through pregnancy without impeding the growth of the fetus. Now for a closer look at just how safe exercising is for both mother and child.

Safety Concerns

There is a lot of misinformation out there about the safety of exercise during pregnancy. With the advent of the Internet, women can find twenty different sources giving them twenty different guidelines for what's safe and what isn't.

Exercise Intensity and Heart Rate

Much of the conflicting information can be traced back to the old guidelines set out by the American College of Obstetrics and Gynecology (ACOG), which stated a woman should not exceed a heart rate of 140 beats per minute while pregnant. Many books and even some doctors still tell women to stay within these outdated guidelines. Beyond heart rate, there is also a great deal of bad information about what kinds of exercise are safe.

The ACOG withdrew the 140-beat-per-minute heart-rate rule in its 1994 guidelines, and its most recent pregnancy exercise recommendations (2002) give women an even clearer picture of what

> ## Limitations
>
> The American College of Obstetrics and Gynecology outlines some very specific conditions that will limit exercise during pregnancy or prevent it all together:
>
> - heart disease
> - lung disease
> - incompetent cervix
> - multiple gestation at risk for premature labor
> - persistent second- or third-trimester bleeding
> - placenta previa after 26 weeks gestation
> - premature labor during current pregnancy
> - ruptured membranes
> - preeclamsia or pregnancy-induced hypertension
>
> (Source: *Exercise During Pregnancy and the Postpartum Period*, ACOG Committee on Obstetric Practice, Committee Opinion, Number 267, American College of Obstetricians and Gynecologists, Washington, D.C., January 2002.)

science has told us is safe. The ACOG says recreational and competitive athletes with uncomplicated pregnancies can remain active during pregnancy and should modify their usual exercise routines as medically indicated. While the information on strenuous exercise is scarce, the ACOG says women who engage in such activities require close medical supervision. The organization also recommends: 1) that previously inactive women and those with medical or obstetric complications should be evaluated before recommendations for physical activity are made; and 2) that physically active women with a history of or risk for preterm labor or fetal growth restriction should be advised to reduce their activity in the second and third trimesters.

The Centers for Disease Control and Prevention and the American College of Sports Medicine say pregnant women can adopt their recommendation that everyone do thirty minutes or more of moderate exercise a day on most, if not all, days of the week. (For more on what's considered *safe* exercise, see Chapter One.) Meanwhile, in a study conducted in 1983, the Melpomene Institute found women and babies tolerate physical activity through pregnancy very well. In fact, the institute says exercise is a healthy adjunct to a healthy pregnancy. However, research has not provided a clear picture of what level of exercise is dangerous. Dr. Clapp says you can safely exercise for an hour. Yet there is no evidence that women who are used to exercising for two hours or more can't continue. What all experts do agree on is that you must get permission from your doctor before exercising and ask him or her to help design an appropriate program.

Miscarriage and Preterm Labor
Contrary to the misinformation out there, exercise does not cause a healthy pregnancy to be lost (miscarriage), nor does it bring on early labor or membrane rupture in women without increased risk factors for these complications. In fact, recreational exercise may actually decrease your chances of experiencing premature labor and giving birth to an underweight baby. A study published in the *American Journal of Public Health* in October 1998 found no evidence that vigorous exercise was a risk factor in preterm labor and found that the more active exercisers studied actually had a lower preterm-labor rate. And starting an exercise regimen during pregnancy also does not increase the incidence of preterm labor. It is important to note, though, that as many as 30 percent of pregnancies end in miscarriage. What studies have shown is that this rate is not any higher, and may in fact be lower, among exercisers. However, if you do have a history of preterm labor or miscarriage you may not be able to continue exer-

cising. Consult your doctor and make a decision together about what kind of exercise, if any, is right for you.

Blood Flow and Oxygen

When you're pregnant, your respiratory, cardiovascular, and thermoregulatory systems are forced to work harder than usual. This is also the case when you exercise. So, when you ask your body to do both at one time, these systems are really put to the test. This is the root of a lot of the concern about exercising through pregnancy: If your blood is being diverted to your muscles, is blood flow being diverted away from the fetus? If you are breathing harder, is that making it harder for the baby to breathe? These and other concerns have been addressed in a number of scientific studies over the years, which have all concluded that exercising through pregnancy is safe with a few precautions.

First, our heart rate and body temperature make adaptations to protect baby. In fact, during pregnancy the entire circulatory system changes significantly to support the new needs of the woman's body and increasing needs of the child. While exercise does redirect blood flow to our muscles during exercise, researchers say our bodies make adjustments to ensure the fetus gets enough blood, too. Cardiac output increases by an estimated 30 to 50 percent and blood volumes expand by 35 to 45 percent during pregnancy, experts say. Therefore, it's unlikely moderate exercise could cause insufficient blood flow to the fetus.

Meanwhile, under most circumstances, if the woman is eating adequately and regularly, combining exercise and pregnancy improves the supply of glucose and oxygen for the baby. The placentas of women who exercise regularly throughout early and midpregnancy grow faster and function better than those of women who are healthy but don't exercise regularly, allowing more oxygen and nutrients to get to the baby. And most aspects of lung function are improved by pregnancy. While exercise doesn't directly improve lung function, it does improve gas transfer and oxygen availability and usage. In fact, Dr. Clapp estimates that training and pregnancy together actually improve your aerobic capacity by 5 to 10 percent.

Body Temperature

Studies on animals have shown that very high body temperatures can damage a fetus. Based upon this research, doctors fear that if a woman's body temperature goes above 103 degrees F in the first thirty to fifty days of pregnancy, birth defects are possible. This fear stems from the fact that the neural tube, which later becomes the spinal cord, is very sensitive to heat. But, just as the body adjusts during pregnancy to accommodate the increased blood-flow needs, the body's temperature-regulation abilities also improve. Further, with the increased body weight, pregnant women improve their capacity for heat storage and can therefore generate 20 percent more heat without raising their temperature. In fact, when a woman exercises at 65 percent of her maximum capacity in late pregnancy, her peak core temperature during exercise cannot even get up to the level it was at when she was at rest before she became pregnant. While active women are thought to be better at keeping their bodies cool to begin with, doctors do advise pregnant women to be careful about letting their body temperature rise too high. It's recommended that a pregnant woman's body temperature not exceed 102 degrees F. Therefore, pregnant exercisers need to dress appropriately, take it easy, avoid working out in particularly hot conditions, and drink lots of water.

Birth Weight

Another area of concern has been the birth weight of exercisers' babies. While babies born to women who exercised throughout pregnancy do tend to weigh less than the average baby, their weights remain in a healthy range. Runners' babies, for instance, have an average body fat of 10 percent versus the 15 percent average. Experts say this fat percentage difference is of no consequence to the baby's overall health.

Pregnancy Fitness Basics

Before you suit up and start training for that Marathon of Motherhood, it is absolutely critical that you familiarize yourself with the basic ground rules of pregnancy exercise. Consulting your health practitioner, assessing your current level of fitness, learning what's safe and what's not, finding out about your changing body, and learning how to rate your level of exertion are just some of the vital first steps you must take. *Do not continue on to other chapters of this book until you have read this chapter.*

This book is written for women who are having a low-risk, healthy pregnancy. Ideally, you will already be active to some degree going into your pregnancy and will simply be trying to continue on with your chosen activity, modifying your routine as your body dictates. For those who have not been active before, we have set out a program for you that can begin in the second trimester (after twelve weeks' gestation). While most women can continue to exercise throughout their pregnancy, or begin a program in the second trimester, there are a number of situations in which women absolutely must not exercise (absolute contraindications) and may not be able to exercise (relative contraindications). See the lists on

Contraindications to Exercise During Pregnancy for Otherwise Healthy Women

Absolute Contraindications

- some forms of heart disease
- some forms of lung disease
- incompetent cervix
- multiple gestation at risk of premature labor
- persistent bleeding after first trimester
- placenta previa after twenty-six weeks
- premature labor during current pregnancy
- ruptured membranes
- poorly controlled hypertension
- preeclamsia/pregnancy-induced hypertension

Relative Contraindications (requiring a doctor's supervision)

- severe anemia
- unevaluated maternal cardiac arrhythmia
- chronic bronchitis
- poorly controlled type I diabetes
- extreme morbid obesity
- extreme underweight (BMI < 12)
- history of extremely sedentary lifestyle
- intrauterine growth restriction
- orthopedic limitations
- poorly controlled seizure disorder
- poorly controlled hyperthyroidism
- heavy smoking

page 2 for both the absolute and relative contraindications to exercise in pregnancy.

If you fall into any of these categories, you need to be under the strict supervision of your doctor and should not be following any of the advice in this book unless your practitioner has said you can. Even if you have entered into your pregnancy in a healthy, low-risk state, it is vital that you attend all of your regularly scheduled doctor's appointments. *Stop exercising and see your doctor before continuing if you develop any symptoms you are concerned about.* While a pregnancy may be low-risk and healthy at the beginning, things can change any time, and pregnancy complications are rarely detectable early on. This chapter will help you to ensure that you and your baby stay safe while you continue to exercise in your pregnancy.

Consulting Your Health Practitioner

Your first step before starting to work out while pregnant is to consult with your doctor or midwife. While most of the myths about women being unable to exercise during pregnancy have been debunked, there remain a number of health conditions and pregnancy-induced medical situations in which it is not appropriate for a woman to continue with or start a fitness regimen. Furthermore, even if you have begun your pregnancy fitness program with a green light from your health practitioner, it's critical that you attend all of your regular checkups and keep your physician apprised of any developments or worries you may have.

While most physicians today are up-to-date on the safety of maternal fitness, there are still some out there who lean toward more conservative thinking and still recommend women "take it easy" during their pregnancy. (I've often wondered if they say the same thing to pregnant women who haul toddlers, baskets of laundry, and vacuums around all day.) You may want or need to seek a second opinion and find a doctor who is aware of the current studies and will support you in your desire to continue to be active (if you don't have serious medical reasons for not exercising).

It's important that you don't just ignore an unsupportive doctor's advice and "go it alone." You need to have a health practitioner who knows what you are doing and can help guide you. Your health and the health of your baby could be compromised if you exercise and don't have a medical professional who knows about it. So be smart: Find a doctor or midwife who is willing to support your desire to exercise.

Assessing Current Fitness

The number one indicator of how much exercise you can do while pregnant is how much exercise you did when you weren't. Ideally, you will simply be continuing your current exercise regimen until your body tells you to start slowing down. Again, if you haven't been active prior to becoming pregnant, you have to wait until the second trimester to begin. Experts suggest nonexercisers wait until the second trimester to ensure viability of the pregnancy. While there is no evidence to suggest exercise can cause miscarriage—and there is actually some evidence to suggest active women have lower rates of miscarriage—many doctors prefer to err on the side of caution when it comes to women who have not been active prior to pregnancy and whose bodies, therefore, are not accustomed to the exertion. That said, the best way for your fitness to be properly assessed, and thereby to determine how much exercise you can safely do, is to see your doctor and discuss your plans. Some questions you may want to discuss with your doctor include:

- ☐ Have you ever had a miscarriage in an earlier pregnancy?
- ☐ Have you had other pregnancy complications?

- ☐ Are you experiencing any significant fatigue?
- ☐ Have you had any unexplained faintness or dizziness?
- ☐ Have you had any sudden swelling of your hands or feet?
- ☐ Have you had any unexplained headaches?

You and your health practitioner need to consider these and a number of other questions prior to working out in pregnancy to ensure that you do not fall into any of the categories that would make it inappropriate for you to exercise. Be sure to report any changes in how you feel to your doctor or midwife in case they may have some bearing on your ability to exercise safely.

What's Considered Safe?

So, what's considered safe? Misinformation abounds about just what a pregnant woman can do and what she can't.

How Long? How Often?

Studies have found that pregnant women can safely continue to exercise at their current level but would do well to avoid all-out effort or serious competition. As for how long you can exercise during each session, pregnancy exercise expert Dr. James Clapp says it depends on what you did prior to pregnancy. However, as science has yet to determine the safety of working out for longer than an hour, most experts agree it's best to keep your workout to forty-five minutes or less, including your warm-up and cool-down periods. New exercisers need to keep their workouts to thirty minutes.

It is recommended that women exercise at least three times a week. If you are engaging in a moderate activity, like walking or swimming, you are encouraged to exercise on most, if not all, days of the week. However, if you are engaging in a more intense workout, like running or aerobics, limit your workouts to four per week.

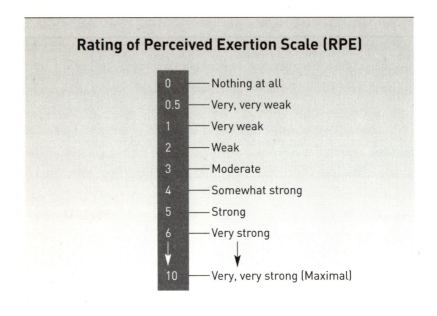

How Hard?

As for intensity, this is not the time for all-out effort. Avoid competing with anybody else or pushing yourself in any way. While the intensity of pregnancy workouts was once monitored by heart-rate increases, experts now say you are better off not monitoring your heart rate during pregnancy unless you have been and plan to do it all the time, as it tends not to be a reliable measure of intensity during pregnancy. It's better to follow the Rating of Perceived Exertion Scale (see above), which allows you to subjectively determine how hard you feel you are working. Keep your exertion in the "moderate" to "somewhat strong" (3–4) range during pregnancy.

Another great way to make sure you are not overexerting yourself is to do the talk test. It involves simply making sure that you can carry on a conversation comfortably the entire time you are working out. If you find you cannot, it's time to slow down and take it easier.

While you can actually end up improving your strength and endurance by working out during pregnancy (due to the increased demands of the pregnancy), stay focused on maintaining your level of fitness, not significantly improving on it. However, those who haven't been active before will see marked health improvements after becoming active.

What Exercises?

Women can safely continue with most exercises throughout pregnancy, with a few exceptions. The biggest concern here is whether the sport is likely to cause some sort of abdominal trauma through contact with other people or by falling. Therefore, it's not recommended that pregnant women participate in aggressive sports like ice hockey, soccer, and basketball. Additionally, sports like horseback riding, gymnastics, downhill skiing, and vigorous racket sports pose a greater risk of falling. Scuba diving is off limits as well, as is exertion at altitudes above 6,000 feet. Pregnancy is not the time to participate in any mid- to long-distance competitive events either. Finally, avoid engaging in any prolonged standing, including the standing you must do in some poses in regular yoga (as opposed to pregnancy yoga). Running, walking, cycling (indoor or outdoor), swimming, and aerobics, how-

When to Stop Exercising

- excessive shortness of breath
- trouble breathing before exertion
- headache
- chest pain
- regular, mild, or painful uterine contractions (more than four contractions per hour)
- muscle weakness
- calf pain or swelling
- vaginal bleeding
- any gush of fluid from vaginal membranes
- dizziness or faintness
- decreased fetal movement
- if the baby doesn't move in the thirty minutes after exercise

ever, are all safe during pregnancy. Check with your doctor if there is an activity you would like to participate in but are not sure of its safety.

Beginners
For pregnant women just starting to exercise for the first time, Dr. Clapp recommends a walking regimen of twenty to thirty minutes, three to four times a week. "They can begin as soon as viability [of the pregnancy] is established," says Clapp. For safety, experts suggest you wait until the thirteenth week to begin an exercise program other than walking if you haven't been exercising regularly in the three months leading up to your pregnancy. And remember, don't try to make up for lost time; don't exercise in an attempt to lose excess weight you may feel you have already gained. Exercising now is simply about keeping healthy and strong and limiting any additional excess weight gain.

A Caution
A big no-no in pregnancy exercise is anything that requires lying on your back after the middle of the second trimester. Doing so can cause something called supine hypotensive syndrome, where the weight of the baby and uterus lies on the vena cava vein, preventing normal circulation of blood back to your heart. This can lead to a drop in blood pressure with decreased blood flow to vital organs—including your uterus and, therefore, the baby. Avoid lying in this position for more than five minutes at a time. If you feel faint, roll over and rest and contact your doctor.

Your Changing Body
It's a good idea to have a basic understanding of the changes occurring in your body before you exercise during pregnancy. This

Pregnancy Exercise Do's and Don'ts

Do's

- Do stop immediately if you are light-headed or can't catch your breath.
- Do drink plenty of fluids, dress appropriately, and exercise in cool conditions to avoid overheating.
- Do rest one hour for every hour of exercise.
- Do eat properly and increase your diet by 300 calories per day.
- Do get up from lying down by rolling onto your side, then onto all fours.
- Do choose workout routes and locations with bathrooms.
- Do spend ten minutes warming up and ten minutes cooling down.

Don'ts

- Don't exercise in temperatures above 85 degrees F.
- Don't do anything that could cause any kind of abdominal trauma.
- Don't exercise on your back after the middle of the second trimester.
- Don't raise both legs at any time.
- Don't do single leg raises unless your abdominal muscles are already very strong.
- Don't assume positions that hollow out your lower back, allowing your belly to hang forward.
- Don't stand in one spot for long periods.
- Don't exercise to exhaustion.
- Don't do exercises that could cause you to lose balance.
- Don't hold your breath while exercising (can cause a stressful increase in blood pressure).

will help you to understand where any aches and pains may be coming from and help you to make the proper accommodations to exercise.

First Trimester (1–12 weeks)
- The embryo nestles into the uterine wall and starts its rapid growth.
- You feel tired and are prone to headaches.
- You may have sore breasts, nausea, and a frequent need to urinate.
- You may feel light-headed.
- Your blood volume increases.
- You may or may not have a bit of belly showing.
- By the end of the first trimester, your baby will be 2 ½ inches long and weigh a little over an ounce, with tooth buds and soft nails already formed and a heartbeat that can be heard with a special instrument.

Second Trimester (13–24 weeks)
- Nausea and exhaustion usually start to lessen.
- Your appetite increases.
- You may notice your weight gain now as your thighs fill out, your buttocks widen, and your arms thicken in response to increasing pregnancy hormone levels.
- You will likely have a considerable belly showing by the end of the second trimester.
- You will be able to feel the baby move.
- You may find your balance and center of gravity starting to change.
- Your breasts are larger now; you may need a maternity bra.

- By the end of the second trimester, the baby will be 11–14 inches long and weigh 1 ½ pounds and may be able to survive if born.

Third Trimester (25–40 weeks)
- Any muscle weakness will start to show itself now, particularly in your abdominals and upper and lower back.
- Your ankles and feet may swell.
- Your bowels become displaced.
- You may suffer from shortness of breath, pain under the ribs, gas, and mood swings.
- You may feel Braxton Hicks contractions (false labor).
- Keeping your balance becomes more of a challenge.
- Fatigue may have crept in again, and you may have trouble sleeping.
- By the end of the third trimester, your baby weighs 6–9 pounds, drops into your pelvis, and is ready to be born.

Warm-Ups and Cool-Downs

With the added cardiovascular demands of pregnancy, it's very important that you work up to exercise slowly with a warm-up and come down from the workout with a cool-down, taking at least ten minutes for each. You need to give your heart and respiratory system the chance to change gears slowly both on the way up to a workout and on the way down; otherwise, the sudden starts or stops in aerobic or resistance training can cause you to become light-headed or feel unusually out of breath. Warming up and cooling down are important for anyone, but particularly for the pregnant exerciser, so don't skip this critical element of your workout.

Warm-Up

Try to make your warm-up similar to your chosen exercise, only done slower and with less power. If you are walking, start with an even slower walk and shake out your arms and legs, taking the time to let your muscles slowly warm up. Cyclists and runners may want to start with a brisk walk. Swimmers can slowly get into the pool and begin moving their arms and legs around in the water, getting the blood flowing. In the middle of your warm-up regimen, work in some light stretching of the muscles you will use in your workout. Once you are done with the warm-up, slowly ease into your workout. If you ever feel that you need even more time to warm up, take it.

Cool-Down

After you are finished with your core exercise, be sure to take the time to ease slowly back into rest. Suddenly stopping a workout can make the blood that has been pumping around in your muscles pool suddenly in your lower extremities, causing light-headedness. This is what you are trying to avoid with a cool-down routine. As with your warm-up, the best way to cool down is to mimic your core exercise only do it more slowly with less power. Also, walking is a great way to cool down from most exercise.

Stretching

During the second week of pregnancy, our bodies begin to release relaxin, a chemical that relaxes the ligaments of our pelvis in preparation for birth. But relaxin doesn't just affect our pelvis, it relaxes all of the joints and ligaments in our bodies. While our level of relaxin reaches its highest levels at the end of the first trimester before dropping off to much lower levels, it remains in our bodies for several months after childbirth. As a result, we are more flexible throughout our pregnancy and postpartum period than ever before. But it's important that we don't take advantage of this newfound flexibility. In fact, pushing our bodies too hard in this way can actually cause injury. Gently stretching, however, can actually help you to avoid injury while giving you a healthy range of motion at all of your joints, something that is critical to overall health. Before and after any aerobic or resistance training, be sure to stretch out all of the major muscles used in the workout. Gently ease into each stretch, without bouncing, and hold for at least at least fifteen to twenty seconds. Only push into the position far enough to feel a stretch, not further. See Chapter Four for more instructions on how to properly stretch while pregnant.

Hydration and Fuel

Both pregnancy and exercise create an added need for water and food. While your body is creating a new life, your amniotic fluid replaces itself every three hours, and you need 100 to 300 more calories and at least eight to twelve cups of water each day. When you exercise, you burn calories and use up a great deal of fluids, again creating an additional need for hydration and fuel. Faced with both of these challenges at the same time, your body must get the water and food it needs. Moreover, dehydration can lead to preterm contractions and preterm labor.

Take the number of calories you will be burning with your workout into consideration when you are deciding what to eat in a day. If you require an additional 300 calories but burn 200 while exercising, you will need to make that up later. Also, make sure you are not exercising hungry. Have a snack about an hour before your workout or plan your workout for two hours after a meal. As for water intake, have two cups of water two hours before you work out, have another one to two cups an hour before, and have another cup ten to fifteen minutes before you start. Keep a bottle of water with you while you are exercising and try to take in one-third of a cup to two cups of water every fifteen to twenty minutes you are out there. It may seem like a lot of water, but your body and your baby need it. A good way to tell if you are getting enough water is to check to see if your urine is pale yellow or lighter. If it's dark yellow, you aren't getting enough water.

What to Wear

What you wear while exercising through pregnancy is an important health issue, not just a fashion statement. You need to keep your body cool during your workouts, and the clothing you wear can help you do that or cause you to heat up more than is necessary. While water that is too warm can be a problem for women swimming during pregnancy, overheating is rarely an issue as the water is usually cooler than our bodies (and should be when you are pregnant), actually causing a beneficial and enjoyable cooling effect. But with most other activities, like walking, cycling, and running, you will need to pay particular attention to what you wear. This is true even when you are exercising outside in the cooler months of the year when you may be tempted to put on more layers than are necessary.

It's important to keep in mind that once we start exercising, our bodies warm up, making it feel as though the environment we are in is considerably warmer than it actually is. When you are running, for instance, you feel as though it is 20 degrees F (or 12 degrees C) warmer. Therefore, make sure to dress according to the way you will feel once you start exercising, not for the way you feel the minute you start your workout.

It may take some experimenting to figure out how you feel most comfortable in various exercise pursuits. Dressing in layers is a great way for you to cool down on the go or warm up as needed. Another key element in feeling cool and comfortable while exercising is to wear clothing made of fibers specifically designed for exercise.

Dri-FIT™ and CoolMax™ are two brands of this kind of synthetic fiber that is actually designed to wick moisture away from your body, keeping you cool in warmer temperatures and warm in cooler weather. A number of sporting clothes manufacturers now carry maternity lines, giving you a variety of options, from cycling shorts and running pants to bathing suits and unitards. Mothers In Motion™, for example, have a terrific line of clothes specifically designed for the needs of active moms-to-be.

Belly Support
When walking, running, or cycling, some pregnant women feel that the weight of their belly is causing them to lean too far forward and putting excess strain on their backs. There are two major ligaments that support the uterus (with the help of the abdominal muscles) that many women find need a little help when they exercise. If you feel you need it, a pregnancy belt can help support your belly at any stage of your pregnancy. Many women find the so-called "belly bra" can help give that little bit of extra support needed to make their workout more comfortable. The belt is made of heavy-duty elastic and fabric and wraps around your lower back and down around the lower portion of your growing belly. With two sets of Velcro fasteners, you can adjust the belt to whatever size is needed and readjust as your belly grows. Pregnancy belts can also be used under your regular clothing if you feel you could benefit from some added support throughout your day as you go about your usual activities. You can find pregnancy support belts at a variety of online pregnancy fitness sites or through your local medical supply shop.

Breast Support
As our bodies ready themselves for the job of feeding a baby, our breasts grow to sizes we never thought possible. Many small- to

medium-busted women find pregnancy is the first time they've ever had to worry about additional breast support. For already large-busted women, the changes that come with pregnancy make a good supportive bra even more critical.

Virtually all women need to buy maternity bras to meet their new need for support. This new need is increased further when you add exercise to the equation, especially if you are partaking in weight-bearing exercise, such as running or walking, which makes the weight and comfort of your breasts even more of an issue. Therefore, it's important to make sure at least one of your new bra purchases is a sports bra. Depending on your size, you may need to buy an underwire bra or even double-up your bras, wearing two sports bras for added support.

While you want to make sure the bra is supportive enough to protect against possible breast and back pain while exercising (during bouncing exercises in particular), it's important that you don't wear a sports bra that is too tight. This can cause damage to your changing milk ducts, particularly in the postpartum period after your milk has come in. To find the right bra for you, it's probably best to seek the assistance of an expert in this area, so go to a bra shop where the sales staff will measure you properly and be able to offer you a variety of options.

Workout Locations

For your safety and the safety of your baby, give some extra thought to where you are going to exercise. Aside from the usual safety concerns for women while exercising, your pregnancy creates some new considerations. For instance, when I was running while pregnant with my son, I changed my route to avoid any congested streets. While the fear of falling wasn't a major concern of mine, I was concerned that running on city sidewalks filled with bustling pedestrians could be trouble: I feared being pushed into a tree planter or onto a sandwich board, so I felt it was best to move my workouts to a nearby park where there were far fewer potential hazards. Perhaps similar issues are at play in your exercise plans. Cyclists who usually take their bikes to work may want to consider switching to recreational cycling at nights and on the weekends and move their rides to someplace safer. High-traffic times at the pool or at the gym also may not be the best time for a pregnant exerciser who doesn't want to feel rushed. There are a number of safety and environmental factors that may be part of your particular circumstances, and it's important to take the time to consider these issues while making your exercise plans.

Motivation Tips

- Make a promise to yourself and write it down.
- Enlist support of family and friends in your efforts.
- Set out an exercise schedule that works with your lifestyle.
- Anticipate schedule changes and have a back-up plan.
- Reward yourself periodically for a job well done.
- Make sure you keep your workout fun; change activities if you become bored.

Making the Commitment

Despite all of its wonderful benefits, working out is often the last thing you want to do when you're pregnant. At times you are more tired than you can ever remember being and you may be nauseous and headachy, have swollen feet or a sore back, and generally just don't want to be bothered suiting up and working out.

As tempting as it may be, fight the urge to be a couch potato and make a commitment to being active in some way at least three times a week. It may feel like your body just wants to rest all of the time, but sitting around is not the best thing for you or your baby. In fact, you'll likely find that if you do get up and exercise, your times of rest will become even more relaxing and generally more rewarding.

So, how do you find the motivation to stay committed to active living? The best way to motivate yourself is to get leverage; that is, to find your inspiration behind your desire to do something. Think about how being active throughout your pregnancy will help keep your body strong throughout the pregnancy, lessening swelling, backache, and other pregnancy-related ills. Think about the restful sleep you can look forward to after exercise. Think about how the stronger you are, the more physically prepared you will be for labor and delivery and ultimately caring for your child. Think about how being active now will lessen the amount of unneeded fat gain, making it quicker and easier for you to get your body back once the baby is born. Think about the increased oxygen flow to the placenta, how the movement and endorphins can calm your baby, and how giving your child an emotionally and physically healthy mom is one of the best gifts you could ever give. Make a list of all the things that exercise will give you and put it in an important place, like in your journal or on your fridge. Look at it often to remind yourself of why you've committed to being active.

Building Cardio Fitness

If you want to cross that entry-into-motherhood finish line with a smile on your face, it's critical that you have endurance. Later chapters will discuss the importance of strength and flexibility training, but this chapter is geared toward developing your cardiovascular endurance while lessening excess weight gain and hopefully minimizing some of the more unpleasant side effects of pregnancy. What we are talking about here is the aerobic or cardiovascular element of your fitness regimen.

Many cardio workouts can be continued throughout pregnancy, but we have chosen to highlight two non-weight-bearing (meaning your legs are not supporting your weight while you are doing them) cardio workouts, cycling and swimming, and two weight-bearing workouts, walking and running. While weight-bearing exercise has been shown to have added benefits in pregnancy, it's up to you to decide which mode of cardio fitness is best for you. Switching among the four modes of exercise is also an option, as long as you have participated in each of the activities regularly in the three months before you became pregnant; otherwise, you must wait until the second trimester to begin any new exercise. For each mode of exercise, we have included sample programs for both beginners (completely new to regular participation in the activity) and those who are going into their pregnancies already active in the given sport.

With any pregnancy exercise, it's important to keep your intensity around the "moderate" to "somewhat strong" range (3–4) on the Rating of Perceived Exertion (RPE) Scale. (See scale on page 6.) You can also use the talk test (being able to talk comfortably throughout your workout) to make sure you are in the appropriate range of exertion. With all pregnancy exercise, be sure to stop and take a break whenever you feel you need to; now is not the time to be challenging yourself. But remember, the cardio component is critical to any exercise plan, so try to do some sort of cardio workout for at least twenty minutes (not exceeding an hour) at least three to four times a week.

The following exercise schedules are examples of how you can accommodate your prepregnancy level of fitness to the new demands of pregnancy. It is not necessary, nor recommended, that you follow them exactly. If you feel you need to cut back more than suggested, do so. Alternatively, if you feel you can do more and your doctor gives you the green light, feel free to make the appropriate changes. But be sure to take it easy and check with your doctor before starting any exercise program.

Note: The exercise times that follow do not include the recommended ten-minute warm-up and ten-minute cool-down.

Walking

Walking may be the ideal mode of cardiovascular fitness for pregnant women because it requires no special skills or equipment, it's easy on joints, it carries a very low risk of injury, and you can start at any time (including in the first trimester even if you are a nonexerciser). Burning between 200 to 400 calories per hour (depending on speed and intensity), walking gets your heart going and muscles working. Doubling as a mode of transportation, walking can be easily added to any lifestyle and is a great way to see the sights. It's also a great way to get some fresh air, help with sleep disturbances, and combat constipation.

Walking in pregnancy is very popular. According to a *Fit Pregnancy Magazine* study involving more than 3,000 pregnant women, the number of pregnant women using walking as exercise rose from 61 percent prepregnancy to 79 percent in the second trimester and dropped to 72 percent by the third trimester. In most cases, women can continue to go for regular walks right up until they deliver. In fact,

Walking Tips for Pregnancy

- Don't push to exhaustion.
- Avoid excessive heat or sun.
- Make sure you can always talk (the talk test).
- Stay on level surfaces and avoid hills.
- Wear comfortable shoes and, as your feet swell with pregnancy, make sure that you haven't grown out of them.
- Remember to take in 200 calories for every hour you walk and a cup of water every fifteen minutes.
- Carry a water bottle with you.

Walking Posture Tips for Pregnancy

- Stand up tall and straight.
- Keep your shoulders back (shrug once and let them fall).
- Don't lean forward or back.
- Pull in your belly.
- Keep your eyes forward.
- Avoid over-striding (take shorter steps but more of them).
- Start foot-strike with heel and end with toe push-off.

it's possible that you'll be sent out for a walk by your delivery team in the early part of labor; it's a great way to get that labor progressing.

Below are two sets of sample walking programs, one for already active walkers and one for women who are new to walking. While you want to remain within the "moderate" to "somewhat strong" range on the RPE scale (3–4), with walking you will want to pump your arms and move as quickly as feels comfortable to get a good workout. If possible, walk five to six days a week with three walks a week the minimum. Remember to spend ten minutes warming up with some leg swings, slow walking, and stretching and spend the same amount of time cooling down afterward.

Sample Walking Program—New Walkers

First Trimester

Walking at a moderate pace, gradually increase the duration of your walks to twenty-five minutes. Continue at this time and intensity until the start of the second trimester (thirteenth week of pregnancy).

Sample first trimester schedule for new walkers

RPE 1 2 **3** 4 10

	Week One	Week Two	Week Three	Week Four
Monday	10 minutes	15 minutes	20 minutes	25 minutes
Tuesday	Rest	Rest	Rest	Rest
Wednesday	10 minutes	15 minutes	20 minutes	25 minutes
Thursday	Rest	Rest	Rest	Rest
Friday	10 minutes	15 minutes	20 minutes	25 minutes
Saturday	Rest	Rest	Rest	Rest
Sunday	Rest	Rest	Rest	Rest

Second Trimester

For the second trimester, raise your intensity to a somewhat strong pace and increase the duration of each walk to thirty minutes.

Sample second trimester schedule for new walkers

RPE 1 2 3 **4** 10

Monday	30 minutes
Tuesday	Rest
Wednesday	30 minutes
Thursday	Rest
Friday	30 minutes
Saturday	Rest
Sunday	Rest

Third Trimester

During the third trimester, reduce your walk to twenty minutes (or as your body dictates) and reduce your exertion to weak or moderate.

Sample third trimester schedule for new walkers

RPE 1 **2 3** 4 10

Monday	20 minutes
Tuesday	Rest
Wednesday	20 minutes
Thursday	Rest
Friday	20 minutes
Saturday	Rest
Sunday	Rest

Sample Walking Program—Experienced Walkers

Use this schedule only if you have walked at least three times a week for more than twenty minutes in the three months prior to pregnancy.

First Trimester
During the first trimester, continue walking at 100 percent of your current workout time and effort. For the sake of the sample schedule below, we'll assume that your walks now average forty minutes at a moderate to somewhat strong pace.

Sample first trimester schedule for experienced walkers

RPE 1 2 **3** 4 10

Monday	40 minutes
Tuesday	Rest
Wednesday	40 minutes
Thursday	Rest
Friday	40 minutes
Saturday	40 minutes
Sunday	Rest

Second Trimester
It is safe to increase your walking time and intensity in the second trimester if you are feeling up to it. For the sample schedule below, we'll assume a 10 percent increase in duration to forty-four minutes and a raise in pace to somewhat strong. However, do not hesitate to *reduce* your exercise time and effort if you feel you need to.

Sample second trimester schedule for experienced walkers

RPE 1 2 3 **4** 10

Monday	44 minutes
Tuesday	Rest
Wednesday	44 minutes
Thursday	Rest
Friday	44 minutes
Saturday	44 minutes
Sunday	Rest

Third Trimester

During the third trimester, reduce your walking distance and intensity as your body dictates. For the sample schedule below, we'll reduce the duration to thirty minutes and decrease the effort to weak or moderate. Don't hesitate to take a day off or reduce both time and effort even further if you're not feeling up to it.

Sample third trimester schedule for experienced walkers

RPE 1 **2** 3 4 10

Monday	30 minutes
Tuesday	Rest
Wednesday	30 minutes
Thursday	Rest
Friday	30 minutes
Saturday	Rest*
Sunday	Rest

* Note optional reduction from four walks a week to three.

Cycling

While many women who are avid cyclists continue to ride outdoors well into their second trimester, and in some cases until they deliver, for the purposes of this book we are advocating stationary cycling. There is a lot of evidence to suggest street cycling is quite safe during the first and second trimesters; however, due to the risk of falling, the shift in a pregnant woman's center of gravity makes indoor cycling overall the safer choice. Indoor cycling is also the most convenient and safe form of cycling, protecting you from falling hazards, nightfall,

Cycling Tips for Pregnancy

- Keep a water bottle with you.
- Aim a fan at yourself to help keep cool.
- Dress appropriately.
- Keep level of intensity in the moderate range; don't do hill programs.
- Make sure you can always talk (the talk test).
- Consider using a recumbent bike (it can take pressure off the pelvis).
- Stay in your seat.
- Adjust seat height so your leg is slightly bent on the down-stroke.
- Try to keep pedal crank speed (turnover) consistent.

Cycling Form Points for Pregnancy

- As your belly grows, be sure keep your spine straight and keep your back from arching.
- Raise your handlebar stem up as far as you can; raise it in increments.
- Experiment with your seat tilt to find the most comfortable position.

and bad weather. With its non-weight-bearing nature, cycling will allow you to continue to challenge yourself with a good cardio workout without any unneeded stress on your joints and ligaments. Dr. Elizabeth Joy says cycling in pregnancy is a great nonimpact aerobic exercise. She recommends using a recumbent bicycle (upon which you sit low and in a reclined position) if at all possible. "They are the best—super comfortable," she says. "It's a great activity for pregnant gals. It uses a large muscle group and it's very safe." Access can be an issue, so if you don't have a stationary cycle of your own, be sure to plan ahead; get a gym membership and ensure you fit at least three twenty-minute workouts (ultimately) into your week. And remember to keep the intensity in the 3–4 range on the Exertion Scale. Below are two exercise programs, one for already active cyclists starting in the first trimester and the other for new cyclists starting in the second trimester (after the thirteenth week). Remember to spend ten minutes warming up with some walking and light stretching and an additional ten minutes cooling down after your cycle.

Sample Cycling Program—New Cyclists

Throughout these programs, please note that the scheduled exercise time does not include warm-up or cool-down.

First Trimester
All new exercisers wanting to cycle in pregnancy must wait until the second trimester (thirteenth week) to begin.

Second Trimester
During the second trimester, gradually build up your intensity from easy to moderate and increase the duration of your cycling sessions from twelve minutes to twenty-five or thirty minutes (as your body dictates).

Sample second trimester schedule for new cyclists

	Week One	Week Two	Week Three	Week Four
	RPE 1 **2** 3 4 10	RPE 1 **2** 3 4 10	RPE 1 2 **3** 4 10	RPE 1 2 **3** 4 10
Monday	12 minutes	15 minutes	18 minutes	21 minutes
Tuesday	Rest	Rest	Rest	Rest
Wednesday	12 minutes	15 minutes	18 minutes	21 minutes
Thursday	Rest	Rest	Rest	Rest
Friday	12 minutes	15 minutes	18 minutes	21 minutes
Saturday	Rest	Rest	Rest	Rest
Sunday	Rest	Rest	Rest	Rest

Third Trimester

During the third trimester, reduce your workout time and effort as your body indicates, but, if possible, do try to workout three times a week for at least twenty minutes per session.

Sample third trimester program for new cyclists

RPE 1 **2** 3 4 10

Monday	20 minutes
Tuesday	Rest
Wednesday	20 minutes
Thursday	Rest
Friday	20 minutes
Saturday	Rest
Sunday	Rest

Sample Cycling Program—Experienced Cyclists

Use this program only if you have cycled at least three times a week for more than twenty minutes in the three months prior to pregnancy.

First Trimester
During the first trimester, continue cycling at 100 percent of your current workout time and effort. For the sample schedule below, we'll assume that your cycling sessions now average forty minutes at a moderate to somewhat strong intensity.

Sample first trimester program for experienced cyclists

RPE 1 2 **3 4** 10

Monday	40 minutes
Tuesday	Rest
Wednesday	40 minutes
Thursday	Rest
Friday	40 minutes
Saturday	Rest
Sunday	Rest

Second Trimester
It is safe to increase your cycling time and intensity in the second trimester if you are feeling up to it. For the sample schedule below, we'll assume a 10 percent increase in duration to forty-four minutes and a raise in pace to somewhat strong. However, do maintain your first trimester levels or even *reduce* your exercise time and effort if you feel you need to.

Sample second trimester schedule for experienced cyclists

RPE 1 2 3 **4** 10

Monday	44 minutes
Tuesday	Rest
Wednesday	44 minutes
Thursday	Rest
Friday	44 minutes
Saturday	Rest
Sunday	Rest

Third Trimester

During the third trimester, reduce your workout time and effort as your body demands. For the sample schedule below, we'll reduce the duration to thirty minutes and decrease the effort to weak or moderate. Don't hesitate to reduce your time and effort even further if you're not feeling up to it.

Sample third trimester schedule for experienced cyclists

RPE 1 **2 3** 4 10

Monday	30 minutes
Tuesday	Rest
Wednesday	30 minutes
Thursday	Rest
Friday	30 minutes
Saturday	Rest
Sunday	Rest

Swimming

Swimming is a great cardiovascular activity that seems perfectly designed for pregnancy exercise. It's low-impact, it keeps your body cool, it provides terrific muscle development and a low risk of injury, and it allows you to feel weightless despite the extra pounds of pregnancy. Swimming also helps prepare you for labor and delivery by strengthening your inner and outer thighs and helping you learn to breathe effectively, says Dr. Jane Katz, a former world champion swimmer and author of *Water Fitness Through Your Pregnancy*. "The best part of swimming in your pregnancy is the magic buoyant properties of water," she says. "I call water the great equalizer." Katz says if you swam consistently before pregnancy you should be able to continue with what you have been doing. However, she advises waiting until the second trimester to start any significant swimming routine if you aren't already a swimmer.

It's important to start slowly, stretch all the major muscle groups before and after, and make sure you do at least ten minutes of a warm-up and ten minutes of a cool-down. It's also important to choose a style of swimming that feels comfortable at every stage of your pregnancy, Katz says. Past a certain point, some women find the frog kick (kicking with both legs bent as you swim) can cause discomfort in the pelvis and the breaststroke can cause lower-back pain. With whichever style of swimming you choose, Katz suggests you make sure your back isn't arching too much. To minimize pelvic discomfort, she recommends a modified whip kick, where you keep your legs closer together than in a frog kick, with your knees bent toward the bottom of the pool and one leg circling outward. With this modified kick, you keep the safety of being able to swim face forward and see where you are going while strengthening your inner and outer thighs, but without the pelvic discomfort. Many pregnant swimmers find that by the third trimester, the backstroke or sidestroke is most comfortable, according to Katz. Others find swimming freestyle, or in whatever style they want, changing as they go, is ideal. Katz recommends a maximum of forty-five minutes in the pool, including your warm-up and cool-down periods. However, it's

> ### Swimming Tips for Pregnancy
>
> - Enter water carefully; no diving.
> - Take it easy; do your laps slowly.
> - Don't overexert yourself; listen to your body for the right intensity.
> - Check pool hours and go when it's least busy.
> - Swim in the slow lane, where it's wider and you have access to the wall.
> - Avoid difficult swim styles, such as the butterfly.
> - Try resistance hand paddles and water shoes to help if your balance is off.
> - Warm up and cool down with some easy water exercises, such as flutter kicks and arm stretches at the side of the pool.
> - Wear a comfortable swimsuit that fits.

important that you swim for at least twenty minutes, three times a week to get the cardio benefit. "And you want to do this all in a very, very relaxed way," she says. While doing laps is a great way to swim in pregnancy, aim for greater time, not greater distance.

Sample Swimming Program—New Swimmers

Choose a swimming style that's most comfortable to you, such as freestyle, and be sure to take rests at the side of the pool as needed.

First Trimester
If you're a new swimmer, wait until the second trimester (thirteenth week) to engage in a regular swimming regimen.

Second Trimester

During the second trimester, gradually build up your intensity from easy to moderate and increase the duration of your swimming sessions from ten minutes to twenty or thirty minutes (as your body dictates).

Sample second trimester schedule for new swimmers

	Week One RPE 1 **2 3** 4 10	Week Two RPE 1 **2 3** 4 10	Week Three RPE 1 2 **3 4** 10	Week Four RPE 1 2 **3 4** 10
Monday	10 minutes	12 minutes	14 minutes	16 minutes
Tuesday	Rest	Rest	Rest	Rest
Wednesday	10 minutes	12 minutes	14 minutes	16 minutes
Thursday	Rest	Rest	Rest	Rest
Friday	10 minutes	12 minutes	14 minutes	16 minutes
Saturday	Rest	Rest	Rest	Rest
Sunday	Rest	Rest	Rest	Rest

Third Trimester

During the third trimester, reduce your workout time and effort as your body indicates, but, if possible, do try to workout three times a week for at least twenty minutes per session.

Sample third trimester schedule for new swimmers

	RPE 1 2 **3** 4 10
Monday	20 minutes
Tuesday	Rest
Wednesday	20 minutes
Thursday	Rest
Friday	20 minutes
Saturday	Rest
Sunday	Rest

Sample Swimming Program—Experienced Swimmers

Use this program only if you have been swimming at least three times a week for more than twenty minutes at a time in the three months prior to pregnancy.

First Trimester

During the first trimester, continue swimming at 100 percent of your current workout time and effort. For the sample schedule below, we'll assume that your swims now average thirty minutes at a moderate to somewhat strong intensity.

Sample first trimester schedule for experienced swimmers

RPE 1 2 **3 4** 10

Monday	30 minutes
Tuesday	Rest
Wednesday	30 minutes
Thursday	Rest
Friday	30 minutes
Saturday	Rest
Sunday	Rest

Second Trimester

It is safe to increase your swimming time and intensity in the second trimester if you are feeling up to it. For the sample schedule below, we'll assume a 10 percent increase in duration to thirty-three minutes and a raise in pace to somewhat strong. However, do maintain your first trimester levels or even *reduce* your exercise time and effort if you feel you need to.

Sample second trimester schedule for experienced swimmers

RPE 1 2 3 **4** 10

Monday	33 minutes
Tuesday	Rest
Wednesday	33 minutes
Thursday	Rest
Friday	33 minutes
Saturday	Rest
Sunday	Rest

Third Trimester

During the third trimester, reduce your workout time and effort as your body demands. For the sample schedule below, we'll reduce the duration to twenty minutes and decrease the effort to weak or moderate. Don't hesitate to reduce your time and effort further if you're not feeling up to it.

Sample third trimester schedule for experienced swimmers

RPE 1 **2** 3 4 10

Monday	20 minutes
Tuesday	Rest
Wednesday	20 minutes
Thursday	Rest
Friday	20 minutes
Saturday	Rest
Sunday	Rest

Running

Since I had depended on my runs for my mental and physical health for over a decade, I knew I wanted to continue running straight through my pregnancy. While it's not always possible for every woman who runs to continue on, it can be a great way to stay in shape and fight some of the ill effects of pregnancy. I was fortunate to be able to run up until three days before I went into labor. In my first trimester, my runs were the only thing that really helped my horrid nausea and headaches. In fact, when I was running, it was the only time I felt good, and that good feeling lasted for a couple of hours after my runs. Later in my pregnancy, running helped control excess weight gain, helped deflate my swollen feet, and made me feel in control of my body again—if only for the thirty to forty-five minutes I was out there. I used a belly bra to support my uterus and take pressure off my lower back, but aside from that, I actually felt more sure-footed running than I did walking.

With all of that said, I don't recommend you *start* running in pregnancy. While an argument can be made that you could safely start a running program in your second trimester, I think there are plenty of less intensive cardio exercises that are better suited for the nonrunning pregnant exerciser. If you did run before your pregnancy, in most cases you'll be able to continue. "As long as it continues to be comfortable, I let my patients continue to run right through their pregnancies," says Dr. Joy. However, many women find once they get into their second and third trimesters they just don't want to run. They may find the motion unsettling as they get bigger, that the increased weight is harder on their joints, or that they are just are too tired to go for a run. A study conducted by the Melpomene Institute found 42 percent of women studied ran before pregnancy, 19 percent continued into the first trimester, 10 percent in the second trimester, and just 4 percent by the third trimester. If you find you feel the same way, there's no shame in switching to a different, lower-impact mode of cardio exercise, like stationary cycling or swimming. Joy also suggests switching to an elliptical trainer: "They are great because they simulate the motion of running."

If you do run in your pregnancy, it's important that you decrease your intensity and the time you are out there as your body indicates. And while there is little evidence to suggest running for longer is harmful, it's recommended that pregnant women keep their cardio workouts to under forty-five minutes, including the very vital

Running Tips for Pregnancy

- Always carry a bottle of water.
- Run in unpopulated, shady (but safe!) areas.
- Avoid uneven surfaces.
- Try wearing a belly bra.
- Carry a cellular phone or a quarter with you in case you need to call for a ride.
- Dress to keep cool; wear a hat.
- Wear comfortable, supportive shoes that fit. (Remember, pregnant feet swell and can widen.)
- Don't overexert yourself; avoid hills or any speed work.

Running Form Tips for Pregnancy

- Keep your body symmetrical (no leaning to one side or striding further with one leg).
- Run heel-to-toe.
- Keep your shoulders back, your head up, and your belly slightly tucked in.
- Don't overstride; take smaller steps more often.
- Breathe in through your nose and out through your mouth.

warm-up and cool-down periods (which can be shortened to comply with the suggested total forty-five minute workout maximum). Also, don't run more than three or four times per week.

Sample Running Program—Experienced Runners

Use this program only if you have been running at least twenty minutes, three times a week for the three months prior to pregnancy. If you're a nonrunner, you might want to choose a less strenuous exercise.

First Trimester

During the first trimester, continue running at 100 percent of your current time and speed, not exceeding forty minutes. For this sample schedule, we'll assume that you're running forty minutes at a moderate to somewhat strong level.

Sample first trimester schedule for experienced runners

Monday	40 minutes
Tuesday	Rest
Wednesday	40 minutes
Thursday	Rest
Friday	40 minutes
Saturday	40 minutes
Sunday	Rest

Second Trimester

During the second trimester, you can stay at the distance and pace you are currently running or increase your pace to somewhat strong and your distance by 10 percent. For the sample schedule, that means an increase to forty-four minutes.

Sample second trimester schedule for experienced runners

RPE 1 2 3 **4** 10

Monday	44 minutes
Tuesday	Rest
Wednesday	44 minutes
Thursday	Rest
Friday	44 minutes
Saturday	Rest
Sunday	Rest

Third Trimester
In the third trimester, reduce your distance and speed as your body dictates, but keep your number of workouts constant.

Sample third trimester schedule for experienced runners

RPE 1 **2** 3 4 10

Monday	20 minutes
Tuesday	Rest
Wednesday	20 minutes
Thursday	Rest
Friday	20 minutes
Saturday	Rest
Sunday	Rest

3

Getting Strong

While new moms often sport buff biceps, most of us get them the hard way—by carrying around an eight-pound newborn long before our arms are up to the challenge. Starting in pregnancy, carrying the extra weight of a child puts new demands on our bodies, causing significant changes, many of which can be quite painful and, at times, overwhelming. But by strengthening our bodies in the areas that will be most put to the test, we give ourselves our best shot at meeting these new challenges with all our might. From our upper backs and our shoulders, to our abdominals, legs, and even our pelvic floors, it is possible to get our bodies in tip-top shape for pregnancy, labor, and new motherhood.

While aerobic fitness, as discussed in Chapter Two, does help to strengthen our bodies, we ultimately need to do some true strength training to round out our fitness regimen and make sure our bodies are up to the coming tasks. Building bigger and stronger muscles also helps your body to increase its metabolism because muscles burn more calories than fat. And muscles are the storage depot for glycogen, the fuel your body uses during hard, long physical challenges, like childbirth. The larger your muscles, the more glycogen you can store, and therefore the more reserves you'll have come labor day. Moreover, you may have to stay in the same positions for a long time during labor and delivery, and this can take quite a toll on your body if you haven't strengthened the muscles you'll need. Finally, strength training will help give you those long, lean muscles we all want.

Strength training, or resistance training as it's sometimes called, does not necessarily involve large weight machines at a fancy, expensive gym. For the purposes of shaping up in pregnancy, all you need are some light free weights, an exercise band, some sturdy furniture, and a little gravity. To get the full benefit of the exercises outlined in this chapter, it's important for you to try to do strength training twice a week. Doing more than two strength sessions per week is not advised, but there are some exercises outlined here that you can do every day and, in some cases, several times each day (they will be highlighted as such). And don't feel that you have to do all of these exercises each time you work out. Pick a routine of about ten exercises that works for you, but try to make sure you cover all the major muscle groups. As with aerobic exercise, it is very important to spend ten minutes warming up and ten minutes cooling down before and after your resistance-training session and to stretch out all of the muscles you've used.

One last note: With the exception of your squats and the pelvic rock, stop your strength training two weeks before your baby's due date. It takes that long for the benefits of strength training to truly take effect, so working out past this point isn't worth the wear and tear on your body. Now let's take a closer look at some basics.

Prenatal Strength-Training Basics

Experts say strength training is essential to improving or maintaining a pregnant woman's strength throughout her pregnancy.

Pregnancy exercise expert Dr. James Clapp recommends all pregnant women start or continue a weight-training program focused on their upper body and a strength training program using their body weight on their lower body. Women who have not done any regular weight

---

Strength-Training Tips

- Never hold your breath or do the Valsalva maneuver (forcefully exhaling without actually releasing any air); this causes excessive pressure in the lower abdomen.
- Concentrate on controlled breathing throughout.
- Listen to your body and stop if anything hurts, pulls, or just doesn't feel right.
- Focus on maintenance, not dramatic gains.
- Avoid walking lunges, as these can cause injury to your loosened pelvis in pregnancy.
- Avoid any position that might put your belly in danger of being hit by a weight.
- Balance becomes a real issue in pregnancy, so sit down to do your lifts in the second and third trimesters.
- Don't do any exercises lying on your back after about sixteen weeks.
- Use controlled, slow movements to protect joints.
- If you are holding your breath while lifting, you are overdoing it (decrease weight and do more reps).
- Exhale on the exertion stage of the exercise.
- Sit while you lift weights in the later part of pregnancy.
- When choosing which muscles to work on, pay particular attention to muscles that might be weakened by your particular lifestyle (e.g., your upper back may be weak from hunching and your chest may be tight if you work at a computer).

training in the three months prior to pregnancy need to wait until the second trimester to begin. Women who already strength train (and have no pregnancy complications) can continue, but should switch from machines and barbells to free weights.

Experts disagree on whether pregnant women who have been lifting weights prior to pregnancy need to cut down on the amount of weight being lifted. However, all agree it's important to listen to your body and cut back as your body dictates. With the loosening of our joints and ligaments in pregnancy, continuing with heavy weights can put too much pressure on your back and knees. Lifting heavy weights can also make it difficult for you to stay in the recommended "moderate" to "somewhat strong" range on the Rating of Perceived Exertion Scale. So it's important that you keep this in mind when doing your strength-training program and decrease the amount being lifted as you feel you need to. If you're a new weight lifter (starting in the second trimester), start with light, two- to five-pound free weights for your upper-body exercises or even begin without weights, just working against gravity. It's also a good idea to begin your strength training regimen by the twenty-eighth week; otherwise, it may be too hard.

Our muscles have two kinds of strength: the kind that provides a large amount of force in short bursts, and the kind that can last for hours. For the purposes of strength training in pregnancy, we are going to focus on the latter. We want our muscles to have endurance, not just strength. But to do that, it's important to focus on less weight and more repetitions, as opposed to fewer reps of a heavier weight. If the resistance is strong enough to wear out the muscle in six to eight reps, you are training for power; if you can go for more reps, you are training for endurance. The exercises in this chapter will have you doing more reps at a lower resistance.

Now, let's learn more about which muscles we want to strengthen and how. (See pages 46–47 for muscular diagrams.)

Deep Abdominal Muscle (Transverse Abdominis)

The transverse abdominis is a key muscle in helping to push out your baby. Lying beneath your rectus abdominis and your obliques, the transverse acts like a corset straight around your abdomen. Strengthen this muscle and you not only improve your pushing ability come labor day but get your waist and firm belly back sooner.

Superficial Abdominal Muscles (Rectus Abdominis and Obliques)

The main function of these top two layers of abdominal muscle, supporting your lower back, becomes increasingly important during pregnancy. Strong rectus muscles (which bear much of the weight of the baby as it grows) and oblique muscles will help backache during pregnancy and give you power and support during labor. Strengthened abdominal muscles during pregnancy will also return to their "old selves" sooner postpartum and give your lower back more support in those hard days of early motherhood.

Pelvic Floor Muscles

Next to the transverse muscle, your pelvic floor muscles are the most critical during labor and delivery. Having control of these muscles is a huge benefit while trying to bring the baby down the birth canal. (Strengthening the pelvic floor muscles will be discussed further in Chapter Five.) When these muscles get stretched out and weakened during delivery, many women develop urinary incontinence and other problems in early motherhood and beyond. So it's essential that you try to keep these muscles strong and rehabilitate them after delivery.

Lower Back Muscles (Spinal Erectors, Latissimus)

Lower back muscle strength is central to avoiding backache during pregnancy and helping support your entire body during labor and

Key Endurance Muscles Used in Pregnancy and Labor and Delivery: Front View

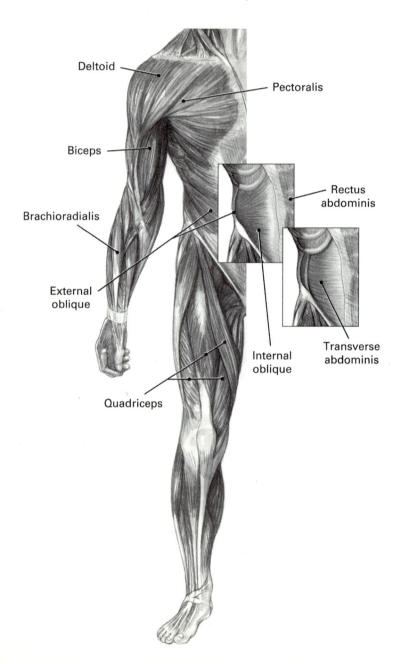

Key Endurance Muscles Used in Pregnancy and Labor and Delivery: Back View

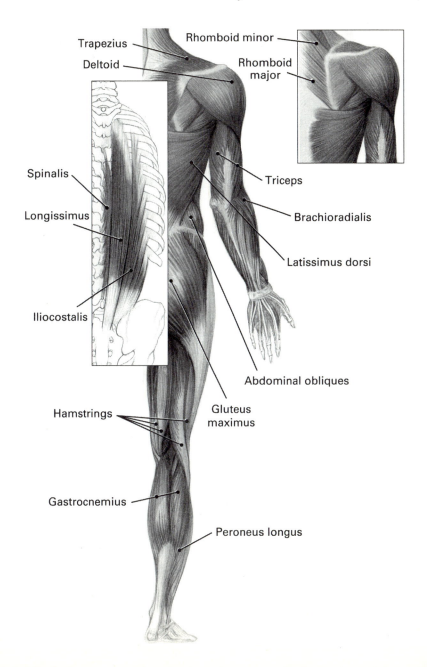

delivery. Keeping these muscles toned can help stop muscle backache from adding to the pain of labor. Considering all the lifting, carrying, and leaning over required in an infant's care, these muscles are also called in to do some hard work once the baby is born.

Upper Back Muscles (Rhomboids, Trapezius, Latissimus)
The postural changes associated with pregnancy put our upper backs to the test. As our pelvis tilts forward with the weight of the baby and our lower backs hyperextend, our upper backs compensate by rounding out as our shoulders rotate inward. These upper back muscles ultimately get overstretched just as they are about to be needed most—in early motherhood. This is one of the main causes of back pain after the baby is born. Strengthening these muscles is therefore crucial to our being able to hold our children without pain.

Legs (Quadriceps, Hamstrings, Calves)
Walking, squatting, kneeling, leaning. The many and varied positions women find comfort in during labor and delivery require a great deal of muscle support from below the waist. Well-trained and stretched quads, hamstrings, and calves can help a pregnant woman feel strong in any position she needs. Meanwhile, stronger legs can give a pregnant woman needed support as her weight increases and give new moms some added support during all that pacing of the halls with baby at night.

Arms (Biceps, Triceps, Brachioradialis, Deltoids)
Holding onto birthing bars, your partner's shoulder, or even the side of your bed can be surprisingly hard after several hours of labor. Strong arms can therefore be a great asset during labor and delivery. Arm strength also becomes essential once you've been handed your baby and, during early motherhood, your arms are really put to the

test. Strengthening your arm muscles beforehand can help prevent a wide variety of overuse-related injuries from which many new moms suffer as a result of their arms not being up to the task.

Equipment You'll Need
Before you begin your strength training, it's a good idea to gather the equipment you'll need. For the upper body exercises, I recommend two 2- to 5-pound handheld free weights. You can use unopened cans of soup or any other item that has some weight to it to start. Beginners may even wish to start with no weights at all and work up from there. An exercise mat, preferably a thin one like those used in yoga, can also be very helpful. It can protect and comfort your knees, hands, and any other body parts touching the ground. While you are standing, the mat can give you extra cushioning beneath your feet, which can benefit your entire skeleton. Pillows for cushioning and supporting your head, neck, and legs in various poses are also helpful. For many of the exercises, it is also necessary to have a chair or other supportive structure to hold onto for balance. For the more challenging exercises requiring your body weight be supported, be sure to use doorknobs or heavy furniture. Some exercises can also be done with an exercise band, a long strip of elastic rubber that you can find at your local sporting goods shop or medical supply outlet.

Getting Stronger

Learning to Squat
The ability to squat or rest on our "hams" (hamstrings) is something many in the Western world could stand to relearn. People in many other countries around the world still squat regularly throughout their day, not just when plumbing conditions require it! This ability, to get down low, with your feet flat on the ground, balancing com-

fortably, can be a great asset during labor and delivery. It is arguably the ideal laboring position, allowing your pelvis to open up by an additional 20 to 30 percent, helping your baby to descend into the birth canal, speeding labor, and reducing back pain. During pregnancy, squatting can also improve your flexibility, ease back pain, and decrease constipation. This position allows your body weight to be comfortably supported by your thighs while putting gravity on your side during labor. The squatting position also makes it easier for you to relax your pelvic floor muscles during delivery and may reduce vaginal tearing and the need for an episiotomy (incision).

Practicing squats will strengthen your knees, quads, lower back, and abdominals in preparation for labor. Unfortunately, many Western women have never done it and therefore find it quite difficult, if not impossible, when labor comes. Learning this age-old, lost pose can be a great advantage to a woman preparing for labor.

Squatting Tips

- You can start practicing squatting by sitting in the squatting position on a short and stable stool, box, or stack of books while holding onto a chair.
- You may want to wear shoes with a bit of a wedge heel or place a rolled towel under your heels, if keeping your feet flat is difficult at first.
- You can also practice your pelvic floor exercises in this position.
- Keeping your feet flat on the floor can be quite difficult at first if your calves are tight, as most people's tend to be. Try to bring your heels as low to the ground as possible when you start practicing your squats and, in the meantime, work on the calf stretches outlined in Chapter Four.

SQUATS

Do not practice squatting if you have any knee, back, hip, or ankle problems. Stop immediately if you experience pain beyond burning in your muscles.

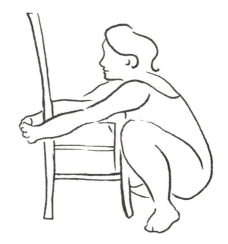

1) Start by finding a solid, heavy piece of furniture that you can hold onto and will support your weight. A doorknob or partner works quite well for this too.
2) Wearing loose clothing, stand about two feet from your supporting device with your feet shoulder-width apart. Let your knees move apart as far as is comfortable.
3) With your feet flat on the ground, slowly bend your knees and lower yourself down into the squatting position.
4) Try not to allow your feet to roll in on your arches. Once in position, don't bounce.
5) Keep your arms as straight as you can, keep your head up and your spine tall.
6) Hold the position for twenty-five seconds or as long as you can.
7) To come out of the squat, release one hand and use it to gently lower yourself down onto the floor on your bum.
8) Slowly move yourself onto all fours before placing each hand just above your knees as you stand up. You are now ready to practice another squat.
9) Repeat eight to ten times a day and work up to three one-minute squats at a time.

The Pelvic Rock

Next to squatting, the pelvic rock, or pelvic tilt as it's sometimes known, is the best exercise a pregnant woman can practice in preparation for labor and delivery and to help ease some of the discomforts of pregnancy and early motherhood. This exercise strengthens and stretches your abs, spine, hamstrings, and buttocks. The pelvic rock helps relieve back and neck aches while limbering up your spine. Backaches in pregnancy are largely due to the shortening of your lower back muscles as the abdominal muscles in front become overextended with the increasing size and weight of the baby. This exercise helps to elongate those back muscles and tighten your abs. The pelvic rock will help you to bring your pelvis back toward a more neutral position, taking some of that pressure off your back. The biggest advantage to this exercise, however, is its ability to open up all the muscles and supporting tissues around your hips, preparing this area for the baby's descent. Used during labor, this exercise can also help relieve pain and may help to rotate a baby into the ideal position for birth. It's a good idea to start practicing this exercise in early pregnancy to help strengthen your abdominal and lower back muscles in preparation for the strain that increased belly weight will cause. There are three ways to do the pelvic rock: standing, lying on your back, or on all fours. Pick whichever one you prefer and repeat it several times each day.

STANDING PELVIC ROCK

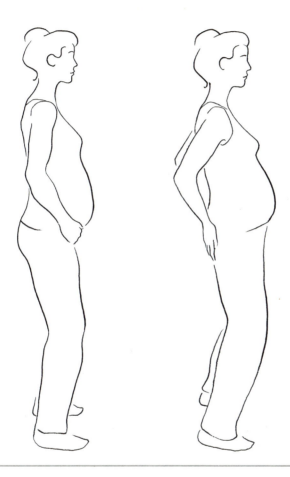

1) Stand with feet hip-width apart.
2) Keep your head up, shoulders back, and knees slightly bent.
3) Inhaling, pull in your abs and tighten your buttocks as you tilt the top part of your pelvis back.
4) Hold for five seconds before gently releasing, while exhaling, and allowing your pelvis to tilt forward again.
5) Complete ten reps at least once a day.

FLOOR PELVIC ROCK

(for first trimester only)

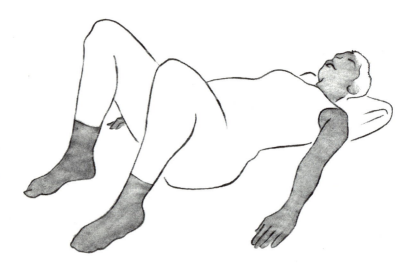

1) Lie on your back on an exercise pad or soft carpet with your knees bent and feet flat on the floor, about shoulder-width apart.
2) Keeping your upper back on the floor, rest your head and neck under one or two pillows.
3) Inhaling, tighten your stomach muscles and buttocks and slowly begin to rock back. Hold for five seconds.
4) Exhaling, allow your lower back to flatten onto the floor before slowly, gently relaxing back into your starting position. (Note: Do not allow your lower back to hollow out. Simply allow your abs and buttocks to return to their natural position before pulling in for another "rock" back.)
5) Complete ten reps at least once a day.

PELVIC ROCK ON ALL FOURS

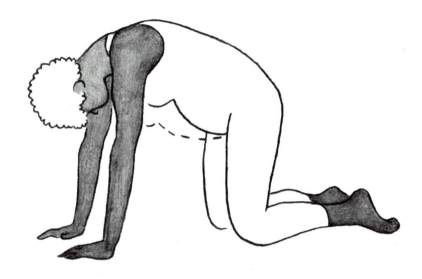

1) Using an exercise mat or soft carpet, slowly lower yourself down onto all fours.
2) Keep your knees hip-width apart, keep your arms straight, and make sure not to curve your upper back.
3) Inhaling, slowly tilt the top of your pelvis back (up) by tightening your abs and buttocks.
4) Hold for five seconds before gently releasing, while exhaling, and allowing your pelvis to return to the starting position.
5) Complete ten reps at least once a day.

Abdominal Work

Since our abdominal muscles are stretched to their outer limits during pregnancy, you may mistakenly think they aren't of much use during pregnancy, labor, or delivery. The opposite is, in fact, true. The transverse muscle is actually the muscle used more than any other during the pushing stage of labor. This innermost abdominal muscle wraps around your abdomen, acting like a corset, and is the one most helpful for pushing the baby out. Strengthening the transverse muscle is therefore very important to being ready for labor and delivery. A strong transverse muscle will also ease back pain and help you to get your figure back more quickly after childbirth. Strong rectus abdominis and oblique muscles support your back during pregnancy and labor. These muscles too will return to normal more quickly postpartum if they've been strengthened during pregnancy. The new demands of motherhood require strong core muscles as well, says Dr. Elizabeth Joy. "If you have a strong core, it protects your back," she says. "That's critical for lifting kids out of the car and so forth."

Before we learn how to keep these abdominal muscles strong, however, it's important to check to see if your rectus abdominis muscles have separated (a condition called diastasis recti). As the baby grows, it's natural for these muscles sometimes to part down the middle to make room for the baby. If these muscles have separated by more than an inch, do not do abdominal exercises and take particular care not to strain your abdominals. Repeat the following test regularly to make sure nothing has changed. Separated rectus muscles can be rehabilitated after the baby is born.

RECTUS MUSCLE SEPARATION TEST

1) Lie on your back, with a pillow under your head, knees bent, feet flat on the floor.
2) Place your hands on your growing belly and very slowly lift your head and shoulders, keeping your chin tucked in.
3) If your rectus muscles have separated, you'll feel a soft, bulging area down the center of your belly below your bellybutton.

BABY HUGS — STRENGTHENS TRANSVERSE ABDOMINIS

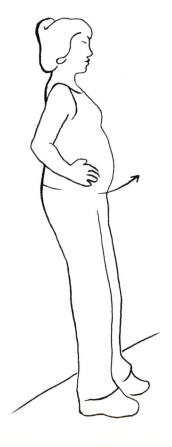

1) Lean your back and buttocks up against a wall with your feet about six inches in front, your knees slightly bent, and hands on your belly.
2) Take a deep breath in and, as you blow out, pull your bellybutton in toward your spine, tilting the bottom of your pelvis forward.
3) Hold for twenty seconds, keeping your abs contracted but breathing throughout.
4) Release and repeat.
5) Do twenty-five reps, five times a day. Work up to 100 abdominal muscle contractions, ten times a day.

SIDE REACHES — STRENGTHENS OBLIQUES

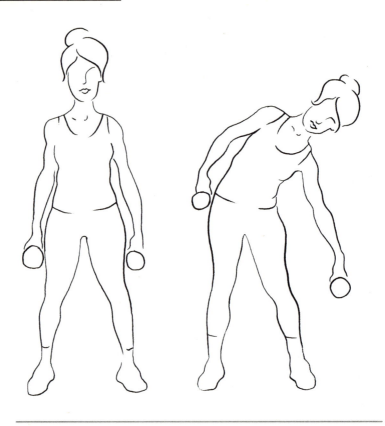

1) Stand tall, with your tailbone tucked in, your knees slightly bent, and a weight in each hand.
2) Take a deep breath and, on the exhale, slowly bend to the left, pulling your right hand up toward your underarm while your left hand stays straight and falls down toward your left knee.
3) As you take another deep breath, slowly return to a standing position.
4) On the exhale, reach down with your right hand, bringing your left hand up toward your underarm.
5) Repeat five times on each side. Work up to twenty-five reaches on each side.

CHAIR ABDOMINAL WORK

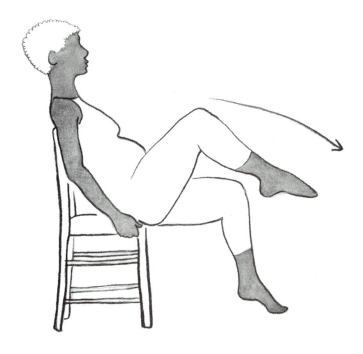

1) Sitting on the edge of a chair, keep your knees bent and your pointed toes touching the ground.
2) Keeping your abdominals contracted, hold onto the chair for balance as you lean back.
3) Remember to keep your spine in the neutral position by keeping your abs contracted.
4) Inhale and lift your right knee up toward your chest.
5) Keeping your knee lifted, use your abs to pull your tailbone under as you exhale, doing a tiny abdominal crunch.
6) Inhale again and slowly lower your leg back to the starting position on the exhale.
7) Alternate legs and repeat eight to twelve times on each side.

INCLINE CRUNCH

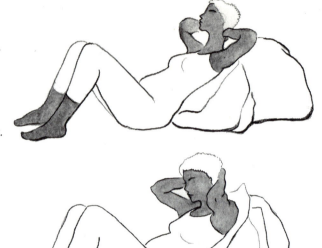

Those in the first trimester of pregnancy can do this exercise lying on their backs.

1) Sit comfortably against a pile of pillows at a 45-degree angle, keeping your head and shoulders above your belly.
2) With your knees bent, place your feet flat on the floor about hip-width apart.
3) Without interlacing your fingers, lightly place your hands behind your head.
4) Contract your abdominal muscles and gently bring your spine into a neutral position.
5) Take a deep breath and, on the exhale, pull your bellybutton toward your spine as you curl your head and shoulders up off the pillows, being careful not to pull on your head and neck.
6) Inhale and return to the starting position.
7) Do two to three sets of eight to twelve repetitions. Remember to rest at least one minute between sets.

Preparing Arms for Labor and Baby

Three days after delivering my son, a five-inch section of my right forearm went numb and I began to feel sharp, shooting pains each time I reached out for diapers, wipes, and the many tools of motherhood. Diagnosed with what my doctor called "mommy tendonitis," I spent the subsequent weeks suffering with an arm that just wasn't up to the new demands of motherhood, namely the nine-pounder who needed my embrace. I later learned this is an all-too-common ailment suffered by new mothers. Due to the sudden, heavy demands of mothering a child, the tendons and muscles in women's arms get swollen, putting pressure on nerves. This can manifest itself in carpal tunnel syndrome (common due to the swelling associated with pregnancy anyway) and other inflammation-related lower-arm problems, causing pain, numbness, even the inability to use the limb.

With all of the focus upon what goes on below our waists (when we had waists!) during our pregnancies, it's easy to forget about the importance of getting our arms ready for baby. From the time that little one is handed to you in the delivery room, you won't believe how much you use your arms. And once that day arrives, there won't be any time to get your arms ready. So now is the time.

In addition to helping you strengthen your arms and prepare to hold a baby, the following exercises will help you support your weight in the various comfort positions in labor and delivery.

These exercises will get results, but arm and wrist strength can be developed in other, more functional ways, too. With all of our modern conveniences, we've stopped doing many of the chores that used to help us be ready for these challenges, like wringing out the laundry. So, why not start hand-washing more of your clothing (some of the baby's new duds for instance) and using an old-fashioned hand-crank can opener? Chores like these will help ensure your arms are up to the hard work ahead.

WRIST CURL AND REVERSE CURL

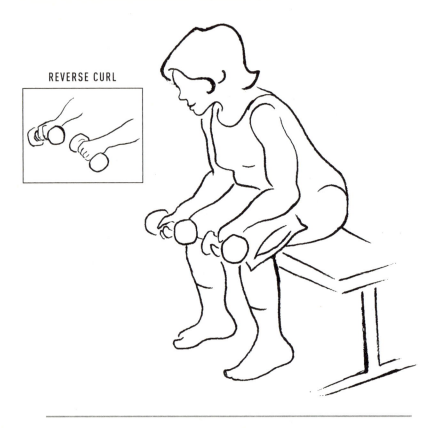

REVERSE CURL

1) Holding a light weight in your hand, lay your forearm down (palm up) over the edge of a tabletop or on a pillow on your lap.
2) Slowly curl your wrist up (flex) as far as you can.
3) Slowly return to start position without letting your wrist just flop back.
4) Repeat ten to twelve times. Do two sets.
5) Now place your arm, still holding the weight, palm down on a pillow or table.
6) Slowly curl your wrist up (now extending) as far as is comfortable.
7) Slowly release your wrist back to start position.
8) Repeat eight to twelve times. Do two sets.

BICEPS CURL

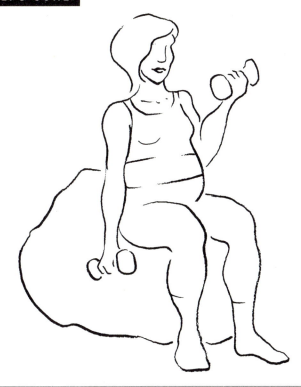

1) Sit on a chair, with a free weight in each hand and your arms hanging comfortably at your sides.
2) Take a deep breath and, on the exhale, slowly raise the weight in your left hand up toward your shoulder. As you do this, make sure you've turned your hand palm-up.
3) As you exhale, bring your left arm back down to the starting position. As you do this, be sure to twist your forearm so that your palm is facing your body, then behind you (this pronation of the forearm during the curl works your forearm pronator muscles, which will be needed for carrying baby).
4) Repeat with the other arm.
5) Repeat eight to twelve times and do two sets with each arm.

ARM EXTENSIONS

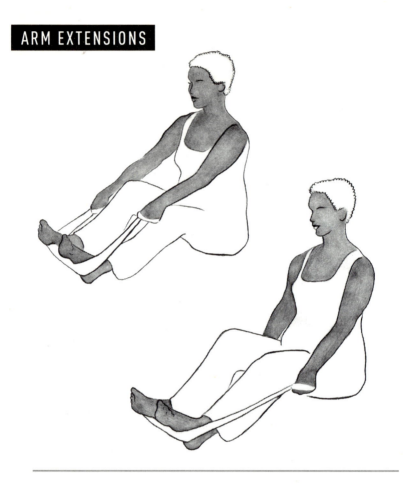

1) Sit on the floor, knees bent, feet flexed with your exercise band around the arches of your feet.
2) Hold one end of the exercise band in each hand, keeping your arms straight with your palms facing backward and knuckles downward.
3) Shorten the exercise band by wrapping it around your hands to ensure you have sufficient tension.
4) Now, keeping your arms straight, pull the band backward a few inches, bringing your shoulder blades together.
5) Slowly return to the starting position and repeat eight to twelve times. Do two sets.

LATERAL RAISES

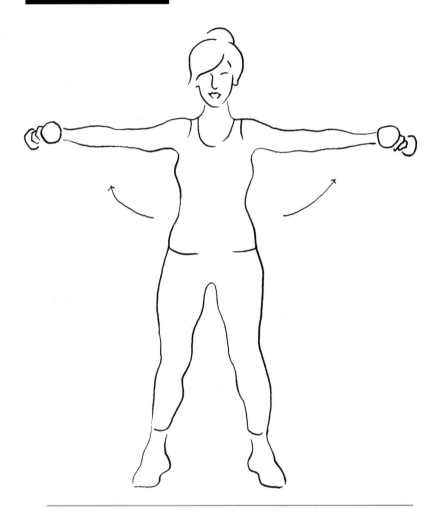

1) Stand tall, with your knees slightly bent and your arms at your sides, holding a weight in each hand.
2) Take a deep breath and, on the exhale, raise both arms straight out to shoulder level.
3) On the inhale, slowly allow your arms to return to your sides.
4) Repeat eight to twelve times. Do two sets.

TRICEPS EXTENSIONS

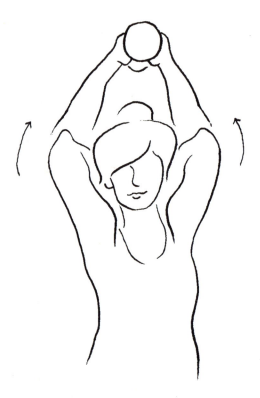

1) Stand tall, with your knees slightly bent and your bent arms up above your head (holding one free weight by its end with both hands).
2) Take a deep breath and, on the exhale, slowly and gently straighten both arms upward.
3) On the inhale, return to the starting position.
4) Repeat eight to twelve times. Do two sets.

When Trouble Comes

If you do develop numbness or tingling in your arms, wrists, or hands, it's important to see your doctor and make sure nothing is seriously wrong. Your practitioner may send you to an expert, such as a physiotherapist, to investigate the cause and give you exercises to do. Carpal tunnel syndrome (CTS) can be very common in pregnancy due to the increased volume of fluid in our bodies, which can press down on the medial nerve and cause pain, burning, tingling, or numbness in the fingers and hand, sometimes extending into the elbow. New mothers are also prone to developing CTS because they usually hold their babies with their wrists in a flexed position for longer periods of time than they're used to. It may help to massage your inner wrist, ice the problem area, and perform hand flexion and extension stretches.

HAND EXERCISE ONE

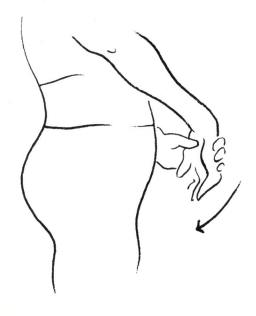

1) Hold your arm straight at waist height with your wrist flexed (fingers angled down).
2) Using the fingers of your other hand, gently press down above the knuckles, bending your wrist down. Hold for five to ten seconds.
3) Don't pull on your fingers, and keep your shoulder relaxed.
4) Repeat two to three times and throughout the day as needed.

HAND EXERCISE TWO

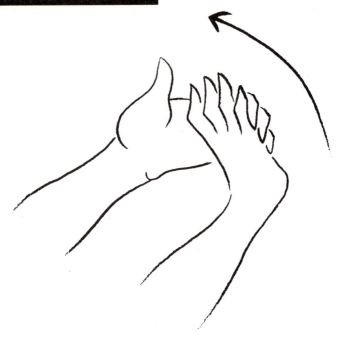

1) Hold your arm straight at waist height with your wrist extended (fingers pointing up).
2) Using the fingers of your other hand, gently press onto the palm of your hand, flexing your wrist futher. Hold for five to ten seconds.
3) Don't pull on your fingers, and ensure that the fingers and thumb of the hand doing the pushing are kept together.
4) Repeat two to three times and throughout the day as needed.

Shoulders and Back

As discussed earlier, your back is really pushed to the limits during pregnancy and early motherhood. According to physiotherapist Shelle Jones, who specializes in pregnancy fitness, the lower back is so problematic for pregnant women because of the strain the ever-growing baby places on the muscles there. The abdomen gets drawn forward and increases the lower-back curve (lumbar lordosis) while the stomach muscles get stretched out and become less supportive to the lower back. As the lumbar lordosis increases, so does the upper-back curve (thoracic kyphosis). This upper-back curve is accompanied by shoulders that rotate inward, giving you a hunchback. All of this can cause quite a bit of backache and discomfort during and after pregnancy.

Carrying the baby around, pushing a stroller, breastfeeding, and diapering can make the problem worse by keeping you constantly hunched over. Therefore, it's a good idea to try to offset these postural changes by strengthening your shoulders and upper back. The following exercises will help you combat pain now and help to prepare your back for the work that lies ahead. Remember, it's important to stretch out your back muscles after exercising them and any time you feel discomfort in your back. (See Chapter Four for back stretches.)

SHOULDER-BLADE SQUEEZE

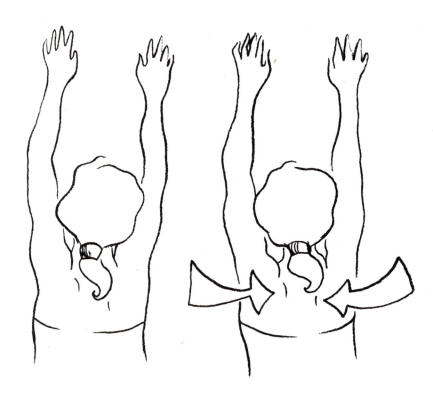

1. Take a deep breath as you reach both arms up to the sky with fingers open.
2. Be sure to keep your shoulders down and back as you reach up.
3. Now, squeeze your shoulder blades together eight to twelve times.
4. Repeat several times a day or whenever you feel upper back pain.

RUBBER-BAND ROW — STRENGTHENS LATISSIMUS DORSI

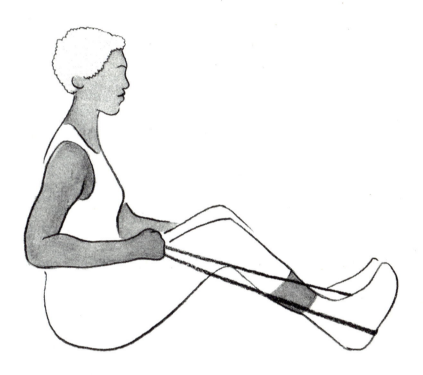

1) Sit on your mat, with your back straight, knees bent, heels on the floor, toes up, and exercise band wrapped around the arch of your right foot. Use your left hand to hold your left knee to stabilize your body.
2) Keeping your body steady, slowly pull your right elbow back by contracting the muscles in your upper back.
3) Slowly return to the starting position and repeat eight to twelve times. Do two sets.
4) Switch the exercise band to the other foot and do another eight to twelve reps. Do two sets.

SHOULDER SHRUGS — STRENGTHENS TRAPEZIUS

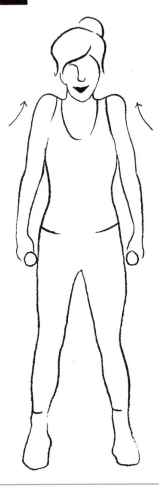

1. Holding a free weight in each hand, stand erect, holding your spine in the neutral position.
2. With your knees slightly bent, and without rocking your body, slowly lift your shoulders up toward your ears as you pull your shoulder blades together.
3. Slowly release back into the starting position and repeat eight to twelve times. Do two sets.

Getting Your Legs Ready

In some African tribes, pregnant women set out on a slow run around their village upon the onset of labor. Most North American women would find the thought of this overwhelming even when they're not pregnant. However, keeping upright and in motion is key to helping labor progress. On this side of the Atlantic Ocean anyway, the way that is done is with walking. Walking, walking, and more walking.

Leg strength is also critical to squatting and placing your body in various other positions useful for labor and delivery. So, it's important to keep your lower body strong in preparation for labor. You are also on your feet a great deal in the early days of motherhood, walking the halls at night and running all the errands associated with having a new little person in the house. Strengthening your legs helps your body to support your increasing weight during pregnancy, too. Therefore, it will be a great asset to you to strengthen your legs now in preparation for the challenges ahead.

On the following pages are some lower-body strength exercises to get you started.

LUNGES — STRENGTHENS BUTTOCKS, THIGHS, AND HIPS

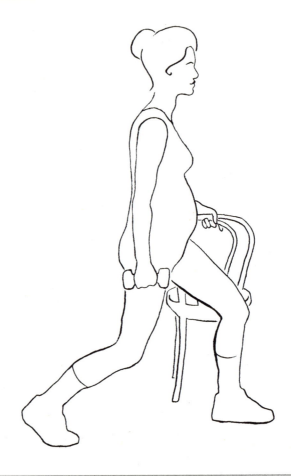

1) Hold onto a chair for support with one hand while holding a free weight in the other hand.
2) With one foot about two feet in front of the other, take a deep breath and, on the exhale, slowly bend both knees until you are in a comfortable lunge position.
3) Inhale as you come up to standing.
4) Repeat ten times on each side. Do two sets.

CALF RAISES — STRENGTHENS GASTROCNEMIUS AND SOLEUS

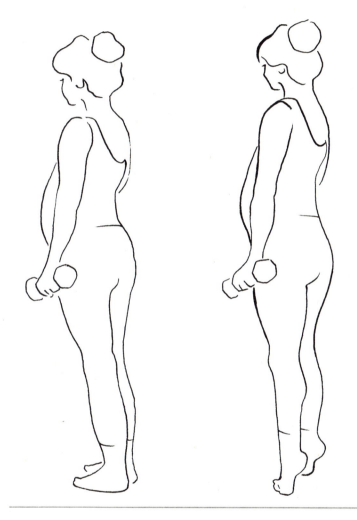

1) With shoulders back, arms at your side, and free weights held in both hands, stand with your feet about six inches apart.
2) Take a deep breath and, on the exhale, slowly come up onto your toes.
3) Slowly drop your heels back to the ground on the inhale.
4) Repeat eight to twelve times. Do two sets.

HIP EXTENSIONS

STRENGTHENS BUTTOCKS, HAMSTRINGS, AND HIPS

Make this exercise harder by using one- to three-pound ankle weights.

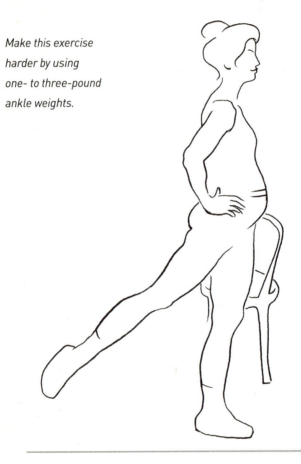

1) With your feet hip-width apart, stand with your left side to a chair.
2) Hold the chair with your left hand for support.
3) Bend your left knee slightly for balance, then lift your right leg up behind you.
4) Now, contract your buttocks and extend your leg back behind you. Don't arch your back or lean forward.
5) Lower your leg back to the starting position and repeat eight to twelve times. Do two sets.
6) Repeat with the other leg.

SIDE LEG LIFTS – OUTER THIGH

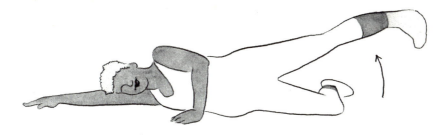

1) Using an exercise mat, lie on your side. Place pillows under your belly, head, and neck for comfort.
2) With your lower leg slightly bent, slowly raise your top leg straight up as far as you can on the exhale.
3) Return your leg to starting position on the inhale.
4) Repeat twelve to twenty times with each leg. Do two sets each leg.

SIDE LEG LIFTS – INNER THIGH

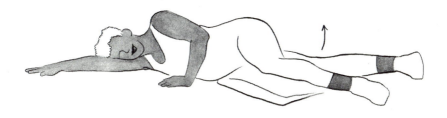

1) Using an exercise mat, lie on your side. Place pillows under your belly, head, and neck for comfort.
2) Bend your top leg and place your foot on the floor.
3) On the exhale, raise your lower leg as high as you can.
4) Return your lower leg to the starting position on the inhale.
5) Repeat twelve to twenty times with each side. Do two sets.

Posture

They call it the "pregnant slouch." If you haven't been paying particular attention to keeping good posture during your pregnancy, you may have noticed your profile in the mirror changing in more ways than just one. As your belly grows larger, it's natural for your body to weaken in certain areas and become knotted up in others, allowing you to slip into poor posture. This is a prime cause of pregnancy backache. The exercises in this chapter can help you to avoid the pregnant slouch by keeping your muscles strong, but it's also important for you to be aware of the features of poor posture so you can correct them as you go about your day. This is the best way to strengthen the muscles needed to stand tall and avoid unneeded discomfort.

Characteristics of Poor Posture

- Shoulders are rolled forward and held up high
- Chin juts forward
- Lower back arches, pelvis tilts forward
- Abdominal muscles are slack, loose

CORRECTING YOUR STANDING POSTURE

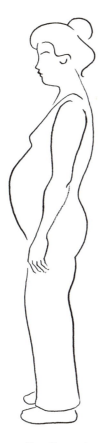
Poor Posture

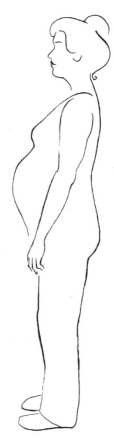
Correct Posture

1. Pull in your buttocks while using your abdominals to flatten out your lower spine.
2. Keep your shoulders back and low.
3. Hold your head tall and elongate your neck.
4. Keep your knees slightly bent and legs hip-width apart (when standing).
5. Lift your rib cage up, keeping your back long and tall.

CORRECTING YOUR SITTING POSTURE

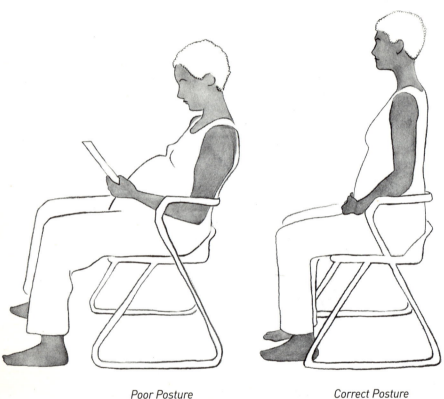

Poor Posture *Correct Posture*

1. Sit straight up in your chair.
2. Tilt your pelvis and hollow your lower abs.
3. Let your lower back touch the chair.

4

Open Up with Yoga

Physical strength and endurance are not the only keys to success in a major physical challenge. The third prong of physical fitness, flexibility, is especially important to women who are preparing for birth and motherhood. While isolated stretches of specific muscle groups are a great way to achieve and maintain flexibility and keep your muscles healthy and supple, yoga—an ancient practice of postures, breathing, and meditation that has become quite popular in recent years—offers a more integrated approach, which is especially helpful to expectant mothers.

The practice of yoga can be quite involved, but for the sake of pregnancy fitness, we will focus only on one pose sequence and accompanying breathing techniques. These relatively easy yoga poses will help you relieve pregnancy ailments and tension while calming your mind and preparing your body for baby. The basic major muscle group stretches included will also come in handy before and after cardio and strength training. While some meditation and further breathing exercises will be touched on in later chapters, a deeper understanding and practice of yoga will be left for you to discover on your own.

Yoga Benefits for the Mom-to-Be

Why all the hoopla about yoga? Madonna did it throughout her pregnancies, and most of Hollywood can't seem to get enough. So what makes yoga so great? Well, the benefits of yoga are far-reaching, especially for the expectant mother. Using postures, breathing techniques, relaxation, and meditation, yoga is said to enhance the union of mind, body, and spirit, helping you to meet the challenges of pregnancy and early motherhood feeling strong and calm. The gentle movements of yoga strengthen, stretch, and open up your body, while the accompanying focus on breathing increases calm, focus, and balance. Yoga poses decrease tension, ensure optimum blood flow to the baby, open up your pelvis area in preparation for delivery, release back tension, boost energy, lessen fatigue, improve posture, reduce fluid retention and cramping, and can alleviate nausea and mood swings.

Your yoga practice can also improve your focus and concentration and increase your energy in labor and delivery. And many poses learned in yoga can actually be done during labor and delivery to ease the pain and help the baby descend into your pelvis. Yoga practice can allow for faster, easier, and less painful labors and reduce the likelihood of medical intervention during delivery. In fact, some yoga positions can even help turn the baby if needed during labor. After birth, yoga can help to restore your abdominal muscles, pelvic floor, and uterus, while relieving tension and other aches.

According to Amy Berry, prenatal yoga instructor at Equilibrium Fitness in La Verne, California, yoga allows pregnant women to achieve mind-body awareness. It helps them to feel less stressed and more balanced, revitalized, refreshed, and toned, making prenatal yoga practice a great asset in the delivery room.

Yoga Do's and Don'ts

While most poses in yoga can be continued on into pregnancy, be sure to familiarize yourself with the poses that should *not* be done in pregnancy as well as learn some basic rules of prenatal yoga practice. First, it's important to note that if you have not practiced yoga regularly for the three months prior to your pregnancy, you must wait until the second trimester to begin. (Skip to the back of this chapter for major muscle group stretches which you can do now.) If you have practiced yoga prior to your pregnancy, feel free to continue what you have been doing in your first trimester as long as you have been cleared by your doctor. Also, besides their health practitioner's advice, pregnant women need to be in tune with their own bodies and know their limits.

That said, if you're pregnant and practicing yoga, avoid prolonged standing, jumping into poses, lying on your belly, inverted poses, and backroom heat yoga, also known as Bikram yoga (where yoga is performed in a heated room). Basically, avoid all poses that constrict the abdomen. After the first trimester, also avoid backbends and prolonged periods of lying on your back.

Pregnant women practicing yoga also need to be very careful not to take advantage of their newfound flexibility (due to the release of relaxin in their bodies) and to use caution when holding postures to ensure they don't overstretch. Pregnancy is a time for moderation, so remember to take it easy and rest as needed.

Breathing

Despite the impressive poses nonpregnant yoga gurus have been known to strike, it's actually breathing, not positioning, that is truly central to the practice of yoga. Each movement is matched with deep and full inhalations, and full and complete exhalations. This is crucial to reaping the full benefits of yoga. As you move your body into the positions outlined below, be sure to breathe deeply, fully, and slowly throughout. You don't want to be breathless at any time. If you find that you are, take a break and ease back into it slowly. Breathlessness can be common in pregnancy due to the limited space in our torsos caused by the rapidly growing baby. Normally, to take a full breath we would expand our diaphragms fully downward into our abdomen cavities, but in pregnancy, the baby makes this impossible. Therefore, it's important that we focus on expanding our rib cages as much as possible on our inhalations. Breathing this way will make it easier for us to breathe even when we're not practicing yoga. Remember: Take deep full breaths in through the nose and slow exhalations out through the mouth.

Equipment

You don't need a lot of equipment to practice yoga. In fact, you could get by with just yourself and a floor. But in pregnancy, it's a good idea to try to collect a few props that will help you ease into the prenatal yoga poses gently, comfortably, and safely. First, wear loose-fitting clothing that makes you feel comfortable and relaxed. Next, if you can, use a proper yoga mat. This will help keep your feet grounded and provide some added cushioning. A yoga strap (a long strip of thick cloth) or exercise band can also be very helpful in easing your pregnant body into some of the poses. You can use your yoga strap or exercise band to wrap around your foot to ease into your leg stretches. A chair and some blankets and pillows can also be quite useful. You can use your chair for balance and the blanket and pillows to help support your belly, head, and legs during poses on the ground. And last, but not least, make sure you have a water bottle nearby.

Prenatal Yoga Pose Sequence

The following twelve poses can be done in a flowing sequence when you need to warm your body up for the other exercises in this book, when you want a quick full-body stretch session, or whenever you're feeling tense or in need of a boost. Take your time moving into each pose and listen to your body, making accommodations as needed.

1. NECK

Benefits: Stretches and relaxes neck and shoulder muscles, promotes relaxation

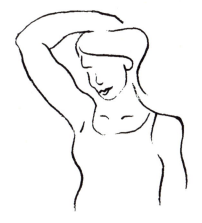

1. Stand with your feet hip-width apart, knees slightly bent.
2. Inhaling, take your right hand and reach up over your head, placing your palm on your left ear.
3. Exhaling, gently tilt your head to the right until you feel a gentle stretch. (Be sure not to jerk your head at any point during this stretch.)
4. Hold this for thirty seconds.
5. Repeat with your left arm, tilting your head to the left.
6. Gently return your arms to a relaxed position at your sides.

2. SHOULDER ROLLS

Benefits: Stretches and warms up muscles in shoulders, arms, and upper back; promotes relaxation; eases body into exercise from rest

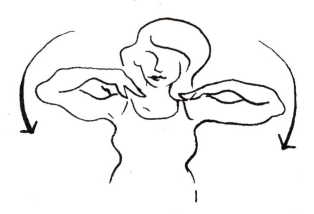

1. Raise your arms up, placing your fingers on your shoulders.
2. Slowly rotate both arms together in large circles, stretching the elbows as far back as is comfortable, but trying to touch your elbows as they meet in the front.
3. Inhale as your arms circle out, exhale as they come together in the middle.
4. Rotate arms five times in one direction, then reverse and repeat another five times in the opposite direction.
5. Gently return your arms to a relaxed position at your sides.

3. FORWARD BEND

Benefits: Stretches hamstring, chest, and arm muscles; invigorates upper back muscles; promotes blood flow

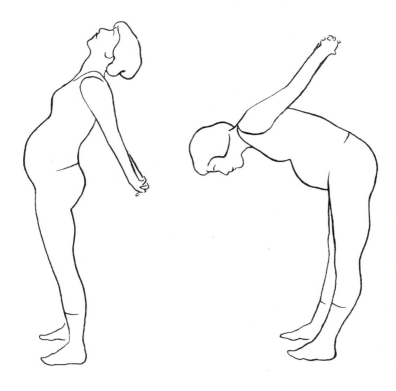

1. Step your feet out to a comfortable distance and as far as needed to accommodate your growing baby.
2. Interlace your fingers behind your back and slowly lean forward as far as you can, bringing your arms up behind your back.
3. Inhale as you begin and exhale as you bend over.
4. Hold for as long as you can, up to thirty seconds, continuing to breathe throughout.
5. Repeat once.

4. PELVIC CIRCLES

Benefits: Relieves back and pelvic aches, soothes baby

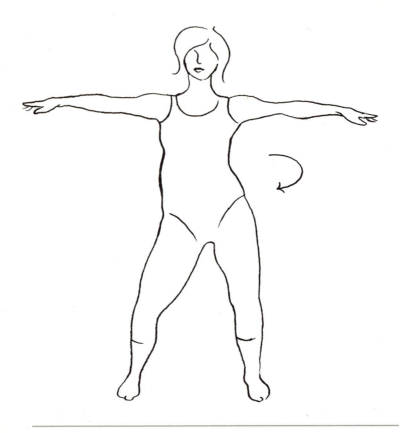

1. Standing with your feet shoulder-width apart, hold your arms out to the side, bend your knees slightly, and dip down into a partial squat.
2. Concentrating on your pelvis, swivel your hips around in a clockwise direction, being sure to tilt your pelvis in each direction as fully as is comfortable. (Remember to breathe deeply and slowly throughout this motion.)
3. Keep going in the same direction for one to three minutes before reversing the direction and going the other way for the same period of time.
4. Return to standing.

5. WAIST TWISTS

Benefits: Relieves tension in your spine, hips, shoulders, arms, neck, and pelvis; strengthens legs

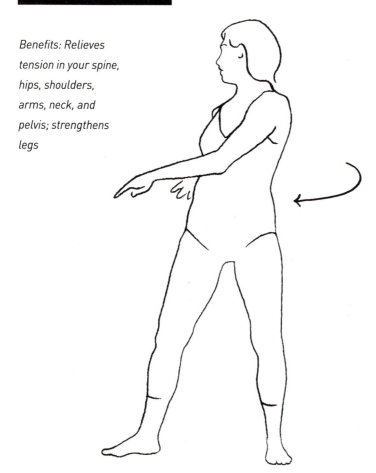

1. Stand with your feet shoulder-width apart, with your arms relaxed at your sides and your knees bent.
2. Slowly twist your waist side to side, letting your arms flop from side to side as you go. (Keep the movement smooth and flowing as you breathe deeply and slowly.)
3. Repeat at a slightly faster speed, doing six reps on each side for a total of twelve twists.

6. SPINAL ROLLS

Benefits: Relieves tension in lower and upper back, strengthens thighs

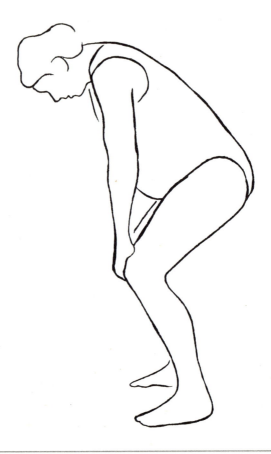

1. Stand with your knees bent, feet about two feet apart, and hands on your knees.
2. Take a deep breath and, on the exhale, slowly start to "roll" your spine from the top down as you lean forward.
3. Once you've rolled down, take a slow, deep breath as you roll your spine back up into an arch.
4. Repeat twelve times.

7. DOWNWARD DOG

Benefits: Eases pressure off of tailbone, stretches the back and shoulders

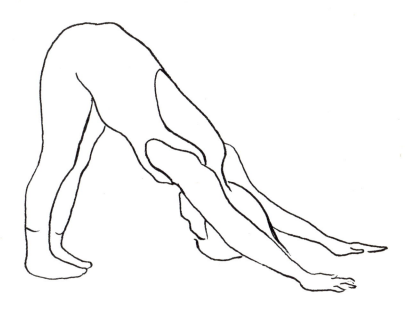

1. Take your time and slowly lower yourself to the ground.
2. Come up on your hands and knees.
3. Now, turn your toes under and straighten your legs, trying to lower your heels to the floor (go as far as you can comfortably). Place your feet as far apart as needed to accommodate your growing belly.
4. Exhale and lift your buttocks up and back, keeping your back nice and long.
5. Keep your breath even and hold for one to three minutes or for as long as you can comfortably.

Third trimester accommodation: Place your hands on a sturdy chair.

8. CAT POSE

Benefits: Stretches back and shoulder muscles, relieves pressure on lower back, strengthens abdominal, arm, and leg muscles

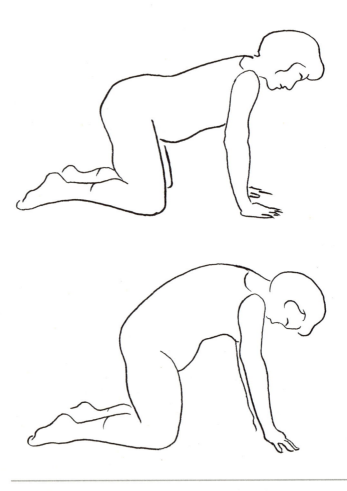

1. Bend your knees and return to all fours.
2. On the inhale, stretch your head up without allowing your lower back to droop.
3. As you exhale, stretch your back up, rounding it out like a cat.
4. Hold for a few seconds and repeat for one to three minutes.

9. OPEN SPINAL TWIST

Benefits: Stretches mid- and lower back muscles and backs of legs, relieves mid- and lower backache caused by the weight of the baby, invigorates back muscles, promotes relaxation

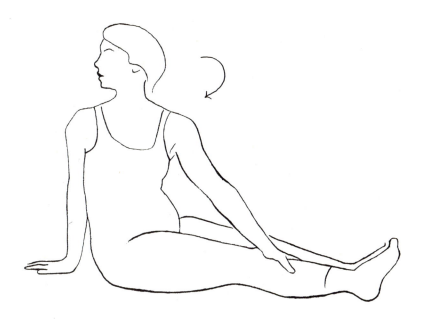

1. Slowly sit back on your heels before lowering yourself onto your buttocks and extending your legs straight out in front of you.
2. Sitting up tall, place your left hand on your right knee and slowly twist around to the right. Go as far as you feel comfortable, keeping in mind that you want to feel a nice stretch in your mid back.
3. Hold for thirty seconds, breathing in and out in a controlled way the entire time.
4. Switch sides and repeat.

10. LEG STRETCH

Benefits: Strengthens hamstring and calf muscles, invigorates legs, promotes relaxation, lengthens leg muscles in preparation for various positions in labor

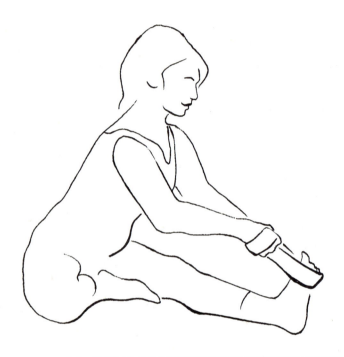

1. Bend your right knee, keeping it on the ground.
2. Place a yoga strap or exercise band around the arch of your left foot and hold each end in either hand.
3. Sitting tall, take a deep breath and, on the exhale, gently pull your torso toward your knee, bending at your hips, not your waist.
4. Hold for thirty seconds and repeat on the other leg.

11. BUTTERFLY

Benefits: Opens the pelvic area, eases labor, stretches legs and lower spine

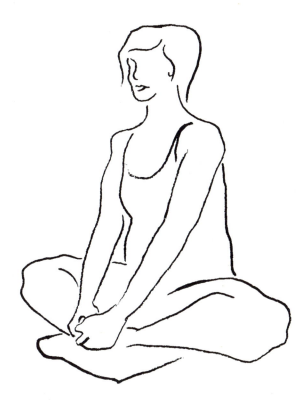

1. Use your hands to bend your right leg slowly and place it with your foot facing inward right in front of you.
2. Now do the same with the other leg, this time placing your left foot sole-to-sole with your right foot.
3. Gently pull your feet together and in toward your body as far as is comfortable.
4. Holding your feet with your hands, gently press your elbows down onto your knees until you feel a nice gentle stretch in your inner thighs.
5. Breathe deeply and slowly as you hold for one to three minutes.

12. FLAPPING FISH POSE

Benefits: Stimulates digestion, relieves constipation, relaxes legs; ideal sleep posture

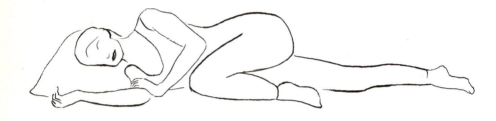

1. Lie on your right side with your fingers interlaced under your head. (You can use a pillow under your head here for comfort.)
2. Keep your right leg straight as you bend your left leg and lay your left knee on the ground (or on a pile of pillows) as close to your elbow as possible.
3. Relax all of your body parts as you concentrate on your breathing in this pose.
4. Change sides when you are ready.

Stay in this final position of the pose sequence for as long as you like. (Some people actually get so comfortable they stay in this position and nap.) When you are ready to get up, use your arms to slowly push your body up to the sitting position, then move onto your knees before slowly standing up. You can use this sequence as a warm-up or cool-down for your cardio routine or whenever you feel you need a boost or need to relax. You can also repeat this entire pose sequence as many times as you'd like.

Basic Stretches

The following stretches can be used to stretch out all of the major muscle groups of your body during your warm-up before cardio and strength training and after your cool-down. You can also do them throughout the day if you feel tightness or discomfort.

CHEST

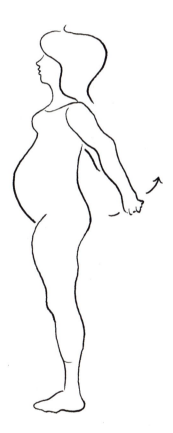

1. Lift your chest, drop your tailbone, and bring your arms together behind your back, with your fingers interlaced.
2. Pull up until you feel a nice stretch in your chest.
3. Hold for thirty seconds.

TRICEPS

1. With both arms over your head, bend your elbows.
2. Take your left elbow in your right hand and gently pull your left arm back behind your head until you feel a nice stretch in the back of your upper arm.
3. Hold for thirty seconds.
4. Repeat on the other arm.

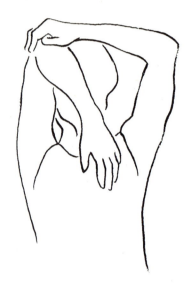

UPPER BODY

1. Interlace your hands above your head, tilt your head back, and pull up to the sky.
2. Lean to one side and hold for thirty seconds.
3. Repeat on the other side.

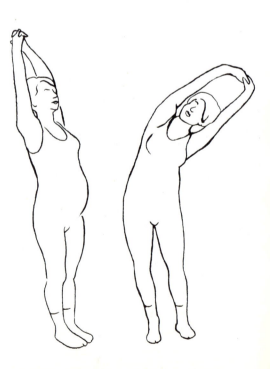

NECK

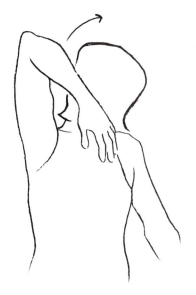

1. Place your left hand over your right shoulder, laying your hand palm-down between your shoulder blades.
2. Tilt your head toward your right shoulder and hold for thirty seconds.
3. Repeat on other side.

BACK STRETCH

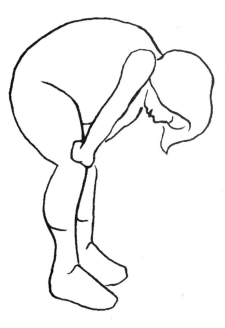

1. With your feet hip-distance apart, roll your head and torso down to the floor, bending your knees as you go down.
2. Slowly roll back up, trying to go vertebra by vertebra until you reach standing.
3. Be sure to keep your chin down and touching your chest when you stand, and hold it there for a few seconds before slowly raising your head (this helps to avoid light-headedness).

SHINS

1. Slowly get down on all fours and ease yourself back onto your lower legs, with your buttocks on your feet.
2. Slowly and gently lean back until you feel a nice stretch along the front of your lower legs.
3. Hold for thirty seconds
4. Repeat once.

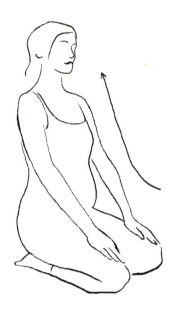

HIPS

1. Standing beside a chair for balance, bend both of your knees and step your left foot out about two feet ahead of your right foot.
2. Keeping your knees bent, slowly lower yourself down until you feel a nice stretch in the left hip and upper thigh area.
3. Hold the stretch for thirty seconds and then repeat on the other side.

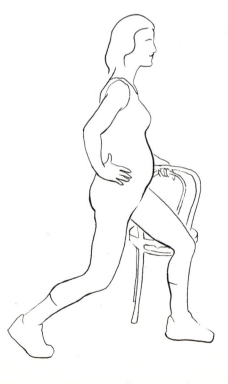

QUADRICEPS (STANDING)

1. Holding onto the back of a chair for balance with your left hand, reach back and grab your right foot in your right hand. Try to hold the foot around the top of your foot, where your shoelaces would be (not your toes).
2. Stand up tall, keep your leg in line with your body, and keep the top of your pelvis tilted back. You should feel a nice stretch in the front of your thigh.
3. Hold for about thirty seconds.
4. Repeat on the other leg.

QUADRICEPS (ON THE FLOOR)

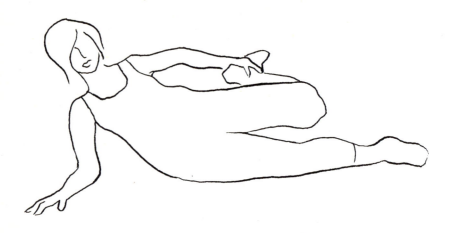

1. Lie on your right side with your lower leg (right) straight.
2. Reach back and grab your left foot where your shoelaces would be.
3. Keep your body straight, your left leg in line with your body, and the top of your pelvis tilted back. You should feel a gentle stretch in the front of your thigh.
4. Hold for about thirty seconds.
5. Repeat on the other leg.

HAMSTRINGS

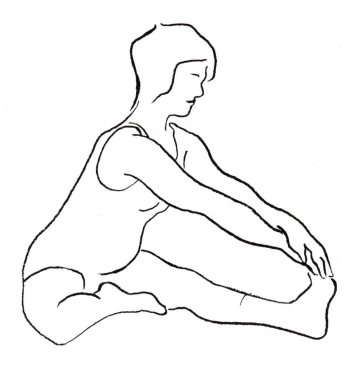

1. Sitting on the floor with your legs straight and about four feet apart, bend your right leg in. (You can use an exercise band or yoga strap around your foot to help you ease into this stretch more easily.)
2. Turn your torso so that you are facing your left foot and gently pull until you feel a nice stretch up the back of your upper leg.
3. Hold for thirty seconds.
4. Repeat on the other leg.

CALVES

1. With both hands flat on a wall, bend your left knee, keeping your foot on the ground.
2. Keeping your right leg straight, with your foot on the floor about four feet from the wall, press down with the heel of your right foot until you feel a gentle stretch down the back of your lower leg.
3. Hold for thirty seconds.
4. Now, holding that same position, bend your right knee, keeping your right foot flat on the floor. (This second stage of the pose stretches out the often neglected lower part of your calf.)
5. Hold for thirty seconds.
6. Repeat both stretches on other leg.

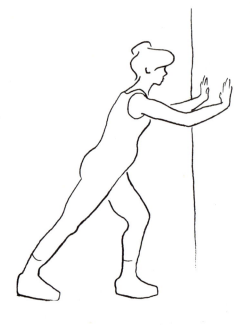

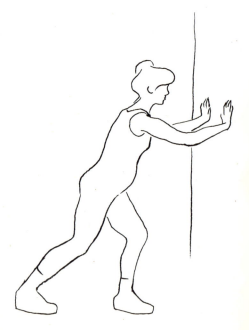

Preparing Your Vagina and Breasts for Baby

Now let's move on to the body parts that really do all the work in this Marathon of Motherhood: our vaginas and breasts. While these parts of our bodies are specifically designed for the jobs of delivering and nursing an infant, there are some things we can do to lend a hand to Mother Nature and make sure we are just a little more prepared for the challenges that lie ahead. First, we'll take a look at pelvic floor strengthening and perineum stretching, two practices that can help a woman in a number of ways, both in the delivery room and in the postpartum period. Next, we'll turn our attention to preparations for breastfeeding, covering such things as breast massage, nursing, and nipple care. Ultimately this chapter will help you to understand the changes occurring in these areas of the body, how these body parts will be put to the test in the coming months, and how you can help make sure it all goes as smoothly as possible.

The Benefits of Pelvic Floor Conditioning

The first thing you can do to help prepare your vagina for delivery doesn't actually involve your vagina directly; it involves the muscles that control your vagina. Called the pelvic floor, these muscles form a multilayered hammock that runs from the pubic bones in the front of the pelvis to the coccyx at the back of the pelvis, fanning out on either side and attaching to the pelvic bones. These are the muscles that hold your organs up inside of you and are responsible for controlling your flow of urine, the voluntary contraction of your vagina, and the contraction of your anal sphincter. They are also used during the delivery of the baby. As your baby grows, it places more and more weight on your pelvic floor, causing these muscles to sag and lose tone; they get further stretched out during the delivery of the baby. If they are left in this state, they will continue to sag with gravity. This can lead to a host of conditions, including urinary stress incontinence, less vaginal sensation and control, organs protruding and causing discomfort, a prolapsed uterus, difficulty retaining a tampon, and various aches in the pelvic region. Therefore, it's important to condition your pelvic floor muscles starting as early in pregnancy as you can.

Avoiding troublesome side effects is not the only reason to work out these muscles, however. In pregnancy, strengthened pelvic floor muscles help with urine control and control of bowel movements, and may help with hemorrhoids by improving blood circulation. Healthy pelvic floor muscles will allow for more relaxation of the vagina during delivery and can help the baby's head rotate when needed. Pelvic floor exercises also increase the blood flow to this area, helping to make the vagina more elastic. This helps the skin to stretch over the baby's head, minimizing tearing and making the birth easier. Additionally, doing these exercises after the delivery can help facilitate perineal healing, and stronger pelvic floor muscles can be more easily rehabilitated after birth. Conditioned pelvic floor muscles can also help both partners more fully enjoy sex both before and after birth as they help make the vagina tighter. And they will help you avoid the embarrassment of leaking urine when you cough or laugh after the baby is born.

Kegel Exercises

Named after Arnold Kegel, the University of California obstetrics and gynecology professor who led research in this area, pelvic floor exercises are known as Kegels. Kegel exercises can be done in a few different ways, two of which will be outlined here. These exercises involve the repetitive and controlled contraction of the pelvic floor muscles. As was described earlier, the pelvic floor muscles take the form of a hammock in the bottom of your torso, holding everything up. This hammock has two "holes" in it, however, allowing space for your rectum in one hole and vagina and urethra in the other. This forms a kind of figure eight. For the purposes of Kegel exercises, it's the top loop of the figure eight, the part circling the vagina, that we want to concentrate on.

Begin your pelvic floor conditioning as soon as you know you are pregnant and continue it into your postpartum period. For best results, do your exercises every day, preferably several times each day. Studies have shown it can take more than six weeks for Kegel exercises to help women who have bladder incontinence, so it's important that you start early to get those muscles good and strong for labor day. Also, as not all problems with the pelvic floor are related to childbirth and pregnancy, make sure you check with your doctor if you have a problem you suspect is related to lax pelvic floor muscles. Now, let's find out more about how exactly to do Kegel exercises.

Finding the Muscles

The first step in doing Kegels is to find the muscles in question. This may not be as easy as you might think. The best way to isolate your

> ## Kegel Tips
>
> - Don't hold your breath or bear down.
> - Try not to let your abdominal or buttocks muscles tighten.
> - Work up to ten sets of twenty contractions each day.
> - Plan to do them while doing specific tasks each day, like talking on the phone.
> - Spread your knees apart or stand to make exercises more challenging.

pelvic floor muscles, however, is to pretend you are stopping and starting your flow of urine. (You may want to actually do this on the toilet once while you are urinating.) The muscles you are using in that process are your pelvic floor muscles. When you do pelvic floor exercises you will be manipulating these muscles, contracting and relaxing, just the way you do when you go to the bathroom. Another good way to find these muscles is to put your finger in your vagina and try to squeeze around your finger. If you feel pressure around your finger, you've found your pelvic floor.

Now that you've found the right muscles, it's important that you keep those muscles in action during your exercises. Make sure your back, abdominal, and thigh muscles are relaxed while you do Kegels. Tightening these other muscles can take away from the work being done in the pelvic floor. When you first begin Kegels you may find it hard to hold your muscles' contractions for longer than a second or two. That's normal. If you lose a contraction, just start again. Over time you will increase control over this area and be able to hold it for longer. And remember, no one will know you are doing them, so you can do them whenever you want.

Before learning the two key Kegel exercises, familiarize yourself with the basic Kegel and pelvic floor bulging. The basic Kegel involves simply drawing up your pelvic floor muscles as much as you can, then releasing and repeating. These simple Kegels can be done up to two hundred times each day or can be done just a few times to warm up for the Elevator and Wave exercises. Pelvic bulging, which helps you practice relaxing the pelvic floor muscles to allow the baby to come through, should be done in the last few weeks of pregnancy, specifically in preparation for the delivery. Tensing or tightening these muscles during delivery will make it more difficult to deliver the baby. Pelvic floor bulging involves consciously bulging your muscles as though you are trying to let go of the last few drops of urine in your bladder. Do this on the exhale and repeat five to ten times each day. Follow pelvic bulging with a few simple Kegel contractions before simply relaxing your muscles back to their normal position.

Exercise One: The Elevator
The Elevator Kegel involves tightening these muscles slowly, in increments, as though you are stopping on every floor on the way up an apartment building. You can choose how many floors your building has, but usually three or four is all most women can find. You may find it somewhat hard to do this at first when the muscles aren't used to it, but with some practice you'll be better able to find different floors instead of just two positions, "contracted" and "relaxed." You may want to sit somewhere quiet, or lie down supporting your back with a bunch of pillows. Bend your knees and concentrate on your pelvic floor muscles. Start by pulling in just a little bit; this is floor one. Now pull in a little bit more; that is the second floor. Pull in a little further for floor three, and as much as you can for the fourth floor. Now, don't just let go once you get to the top floor. Try to release the

muscles little by little, stopping at the third floor, the second floor, and the first floor before releasing all together. Start with ten full Elevators twice daily and work up to twenty twice daily. Ultimately, when you get back to ground floor you will want to include a "basement level" below ground floor, which moves you into the pelvic floor bulging stage. Remember to follow bulging with some simple Kegels.

Exercise Two: The Wave

To do this exercise, it's important to remember that your pelvic floor forms a figure eight around your vagina and urethra at one end and your anus at the other. Start by contracting the muscles around your anus, then add in the muscles around your vagina, then move forward to the muscles around the urethra. This is the crest of the wave. Now, descend by releasing the muscles at the urethra, then the vagina, then the anus. Once you come to the bottom of your wave, try to descend further into the pelvic bulging stage. Remember to follow up with some simple Kegels after your bulges before completing your Kegel session. Start by doing the Wave ten to fifteen times, twice daily and work up to fifty waves, twice daily.

Manual Perineum Stretching

The perineum is the section of flesh between the vagina and the anus, and in most cases, 85 percent in fact, the perineums of women who deliver their babies vaginally will tear. In an effort to control the tearing, and to facilitate the delivery of the baby, some doctors will surgically cut the perineum to enlarge the opening of the vagina, a procedure known as an episiotomy. While this practice is still quite common in North America, it has been the subject of quite a lot of controversy. Many people feel episiotomies are not necessary and are just a way of hastening delivery at the expense of the woman's health. Women who avoid episiotomies are less likely to have such complications as blood loss, postpartum pain, infection, pain during intercourse, and loss of sphincter control. An episiotomy does, however, serve two main beneficial functions: 1) It helps to avoid major irregular tearing, which is difficult to repair; 2) By allowing the head to deliver more quickly, it shortens the time that the nerves supplying the pelvic floor are being compressed by the baby's head, thereby lessening the likelihood of postpartum urinary stress incontinence.

While in some cases it may be medically necessary to have an episiotomy (usually to avoid a major tear), ideally all women would be able to avoid it. Studies have shown perineal massage—a technique used in the last trimester of pregnancy to stretch and prepare the perineum for birth—can help women avoid episiotomies and tearing. A March 2000 study published in *Obstetrics and Gynecology* showed first-time mothers who did perineal massage were 60 percent less likely to tear. Research on benefits to women who have subsequent children remains unclear, yet many experts still advise women to give it a try. In addition, massaging this area can allow you to begin to feel the sensations of birth while learning how to control the muscles, improving your ability to relax them when needed in birth. Doing perineal massage won't guarantee you won't tear or need an episiotomy, but it can help lessen the chances.

How It's Done

You can begin perineal massage any time after the thirty-fifth week of your pregnancy, and try to do it for about ten minutes a day. To begin, find yourself a quiet, private, comfortable spot in your house and pick a time when you are not likely to be disturbed. Take off your clothing, prop yourself up with some pillows, and use a mirror to help you locate the perineum. You may want to do this just after a warm bath, or place warm compresses on the area for about ten min-

> **Perineal Massage Don'ts**
>
> - Don't massage the top of the vagina where the urethra is located, as this may cause urinary tract infections.
> - Don't use oil for a lubricant; only water-soluble lubricants like KY should be used intravaginally so that the vagina's natural cleansing mechanism can work. (The vagina's secretions are water-based.)
> - Don't massage your perineum if you have herpes lesions; this may cause them to spread to other areas.
> - Don't be too rough; vigorous massage can cause bruising and swelling.

utes prior to your stretching session. With clean hands, place a small amount of a water-soluble lubricant, such as KY Jelly™, on your thumbs and the outside of your perineum. Place your thumbs (or just one thumb if you have difficulty with both) about one inch inside your vagina, press downward, and pull toward the sides, pressing in a U-shape. You'll feel a slight stretching, tingling, and perhaps a light burning. Stop if you feel serious pain. Hold this stretch, continuing to press back and forth, for about two minutes or until the area begins to feel numb. As you are stretching this area, breathe deeply and slowly and try to relax these muscles. If you have scar tissue from a previous birth, it will likely not stretch as easily and may need extra attention. Take extra time to work on those areas. To help prepare you mentally for the birth as well, you might want to imagine your baby's head coming through your vagina as you are doing this. If your belly is too big for you to comfortably reach, you will need a partner to help out with this. Make sure he or she is sensitive to how much pressure is comfortable for you. Do this massage at least once a day.

Preparing Your Breasts, Nipples, and You

While we may not always like the physical changes that come with pregnancy, one development many women (and their partners!) do enjoy is the growth of their breasts. Many women go up at least one cup size or more in pregnancy and can grow even larger once their milk comes in after birth. Aside from the aesthetic change, and subsequent purchase of larger bras, many women don't think much about their breasts in preparation for birth and early motherhood. While breastfeeding does come naturally in most cases, with the right instruction, there is a lot women can do to help prepare their breasts, and themselves in relation to their breasts, in pregnancy.

Even in the best of circumstances, the early days of motherhood can be marred by such things as bleeding and cracked nipples, painful engorgement, and insufficient milk supplies. These complications can be quite overwhelming to deal with and often need to be handled with professional guidance at the time. There are, however, some things women can do to help avoid some of these problems, such as checking for inverted nipples, learning more about nipple and breast care, and realizing the importance of breastfeeding education.

Nipple and Breast Care

There was a time when women were encouraged to use towels to aggressively rub their nipples in an effort to "toughen them up" for nursing their babies. The idea was that because a baby's suction is so strong and can cause cracked and bleeding nipples, it's best to try to get the skin ready by starting the "damage" before the baby arrives. That way of thinking has since been put aside in favor of less aggressive approaches to prenatal breast care. According to La Leche League, an international breastfeeding authority, there isn't a lot women can do to prepare their breasts for breastfeeding. In fact, unless you have inverted nipples and your doctor recommends ways to begin to evert the nipple, tweaking or rubbing your nipples before birth can actually cause damage. Doing this in pregnancy can also stimulate the onset of labor, so women at risk for preterm labor need to be particularly careful. However, there are some things women can do to help prepare their nipples and breasts for baby.

- Expose breasts to sunlight and air (helps stimulate production of natural, needed oils on the nipples).
- Avoid washing your breasts with soaps (they can interfere with natural oils); instead, wash your breasts with plain water.
- Don't use a washcloth to scrub your breasts or nipples.
- Don't rub your breasts dry; let them dry naturally.
- Avoid applying any drying agents like alcohol or witch hazel to your breasts or nipples.
- Remove plastic liners in nursing bras to allow nipples to breathe.
- Wear a maternity or nursing bra that fits—one that's not too tight but still supportive.
- Eat a well-balanced diet with sufficient fats and protein to encourage milk production.

Meanwhile, La Leche League does recommend some light breast massage in the later stages of pregnancy, once the risk of premature labor is past. Using a natural oil, gently massage your breasts, pressing in a circular motion and in a clockwise direction. Start from the base of the breast near your chest and slowly work down toward the areola (darker area around nipple). A great lotion to use on the nipple itself is Lansinoh™, the purest form of USP-modified lanolin available. The nipple can be very gently massaged with Lansinoh™

or another oil. If any colostrum, premature breast milk, is expressed during your massages, you can rub it gently into your nipple. Breast and nipple massage can help increase blood flow, lubricate and soften the skin, and allow you to familiarize yourself with your breasts, something that will definitely come in handy when your breasts suddenly become the second most important thing to you in the world.

Finally, you will want to get fitted for a couple nursing bras about three weeks before your due date. It's a good idea to go to a proper bra shop where you can be measured to make sure you are wearing the correct size. This can help you avoid a lot of pain and one very harried, hysterical jaunt to the bra store postpartum.

Checking for Inverted Nipples

After my little boy was finally diapered, swaddled, and handed back to me, the first thing my nurse did was pull off my gown and get me to start breastfeeding. And the first thing she said once she had done that was, "You have flat nipples, so you're going to have to really work to get these into his mouth." I didn't know what she meant and soon found myself flustered, worried, and in quite a bit of pain, actually. I have since learned that 'flat' or even 'inverted nipples' are relatively common. Between 28 and 35 percent of all women having a child for the first time have nipples that don't extend well. All this means is that the insides of these nipples don't naturally pop out the way most nipples do, making it more difficult for babies to latch on. While experts disagree on whether formally screening women for inverted nipples is necessary, it's probably a good idea for women to check to see for themselves what kind of nipples they have before they have to use them. This will save you a great deal of trouble, pain, and worry in the early days of motherhood. If you do have inverted nipples, there are things that can be done to correct the problem, and—don't worry—in any case, you will be able to breastfeed.

To check to see if your nipples are inverted, make a C shape with your right hand, place your thumb and first finger around the areola, and push back against your chest. Use a mirror to look at the side view of your breasts. If your nipple collapses in, you have inverted nipples. A "normal" nipple will move forward. If yours don't, you will need to train your nipples to come out so they can be easily suckled by your baby. Some experts insist the baby will do the job of pulling the nipple out into position, but it's probably a good idea to seek out some help before the baby comes to see what your options are.

Correction Methods
One way to train your nipples is to wear breast shells in the last two to three months of pregnancy. These plastic cups are placed on your breasts and pull the nipples out into the correct extended position and also work to catch leaking milk. The shells consist of two pieces of plastic, the inner piece fitting over your nipple, causing the nipple to protrude. (Note that these are different from nipple shields, which resemble a nipple on a bottle and won't help inverted nipples.) You can begin by wearing these shells for short periods of time, then progress to eight to ten hours a day. You can also wear these shells for short periods of time before feeding your baby after birth. Remember to wear a bra that is at least one size larger than what you would normally need to wear so that the shells don't press against your breasts. Electric and manual breast pumps can be used for bringing out inverted nipples as well. La Leche League also has information about a nipple-stretching technique, called the Hoffman Technique, that can be used to help draw out flat nipples.

Breastfeeding Education
In most cases, sore nipples during breastfeeding happen early on in the postpartum period and are caused by improper positioning and

latching. The best way to avoid this pain in the postpartum period, and to make sure your nursing experience is a pleasurable one, is to arm yourself with information, guidance, and support.

The first thing every expectant mother who wants to breastfeed needs to learn is how to get the baby to latch properly. Take a breastfeeding class, buy breastfeeding books (and keep them on standby), and take a good look at your nipples to try to imagine what you have to do. Taking the first few postpartum days "a little at a time," before your milk has actually come in, is also very important. A few minutes of suckling on each breast as often as you wish is far less likely to cause sore and cracked nipples than long periods. Once the milk comes in (and remember, it will come in—even if the baby can't be nursed right away for some reason), longer sessions can begin. Some other great ways to prepare for breastfeeding include:

- Set up a nursing station in your home, complete with lots of pillows, a comfy chair, and a footstool.
- Post phone numbers of women who have breastfed.
- Post phone numbers of lactation consultants.
- Buy some nursing tops.
- Buy at least one nursing nightgown.
- Consider buying a proper nursing pillow (shaped like a U, fitting around your waist under you arms, holding the baby at the right height).
- Consider buying a sling carrier to facilitate nursing.

For more information on breastfeeding, contact La Leche League at 1-800-LA-LECHE or go to www.lalecheleague.org.

6

Eating for Two

They say we're not supposed to worry about our weight when we're pregnant. "Eat what you want!" "You're eating for two!" "If you could ever get away with it, now's the time!" The truth is, however, eating whatever you want whenever you want isn't good for you—and it isn't good for your baby.

Putting on too much weight can cause gestational diabetes and preeclampsia, two prenatal conditions that can put you and your baby at risk. Gaining excessive weight can also intensify the normal aches and pains of pregnancy and increase the likelihood that you'll have a cesarean birth or that your baby will be too large. In addition, gaining too much weight can cause you to develop body-image problems and leave you overwhelmed by the amount of weight you have to lose once the baby is born.

The weight you gain in pregnancy can also have long-term repercussions on your health. A study in the August 2002 issue of *Obstetrics and Gynecology* found women who gain more than the recommended weight during pregnancy, and who fail to lose this weight six months after giving birth, are at a much higher risk of being obese nearly a decade later. That said, pregnancy is not the time to diet or lose weight. To do so would be unhealthy and potentially harmful to the baby. Gaining a proper amount of weight is critical to having a healthy baby, staying healthy yourself, and building up the fat and fluids needed to breastfeed.

So we can't diet and we can't eat whatever we want, so what can we do? The key words here are balance, variety, and moderation. Seventy percent of Americans eat more calories in a day than they need to, and with pregnancy hormones working to help you pack on extra fat, pregnancy can be a negative turning point weight-wise if you aren't already eating well. To stay in control of your weight gain, you'll need to recognize the key elements of a healthy prenatal diet and understand how each nutrient helps your body build your perfect little baby. In addition to healthy eating throughout the pregnancy, you'll be able to prepare specifically for the big day by carbo-loading and keeping hydrated. You'll also want to continue your strategic eating and nutritional planning into the long haul that is the early postpartum period. Let's take a look at the nutritional basics of eating for two.

Staying in Control

Your Starting Point

How much you eat during your pregnancy depends largely on how healthy your body weight is when you become pregnant. While weight loss in pregnancy is never recommended, the extra amount of calories women are encouraged to eat during pregnancy is not standard across the board.

Many people believe every woman who is pregnant needs an extra 300 calories a day on top of what she was eating before pregnancy. This is not always necessary. In fact, it can lead to excess weight gain in women who already have extra calories stored in their

> ## Your Body and Baby by Numbers
>
> ### Pregnancy Weight Gain
>
> - 25 percent is fetus
> - 6 percent is amniotic fluid
> - 5 percent is placenta
> - Remaining weight gain is due to expansion of tissues, volume of blood, and fat stores
>
> ### Weight Gain by Trimester
>
> - 3-4 pounds in the first trimester
> - 12-14 pounds in the second trimester
> - 8-10 pounds in the third trimester

bodies as fat. Nutritionists recommend pregnant women eat an additional 100 (a little more than a cup of skim milk) to 300 calories (the equivalent of one glass of whole milk) each day, with women who are already a healthy body weight eating the full 300 calories each day. Women who are overweight will likely need less than that, but they need to consult with their doctor to find out just how much extra fuel their body requires in pregnancy. It's a good idea to take a look at your prepregnancy Body Mass Index (BMI) at the start of your pregnancy to determine if you are starting at a healthy weight. (See Body Mass Index and Recommended Pregnancy Weight Gain charts on page 122 for your BMI and recommended weight gain.) Knowing if you are in a healthy range to begin with can also help you to feel better about your weight gain as you continue into your pregnancy.

The recommended weight gain in pregnancy is between twenty-five and thirty-five pounds. Women who are underweight are

Body Mass Index—Your Ideal Weight

What the scale says we weigh is not the best indication of how close we are to our healthiest weight. Our height, body type, bone structure, and genetics all work together to make every person unique. Therefore, everyone has a different ideal body-weight range. The most widely accepted indicator of your ideal weight range is the Body Mass Index (BMI), created by the American Dietetic Association (ADA). The BMI allows a person to calculate his or her ideal body-mass range. Readings between 19 and 25 are considered an "acceptable" body-mass index. Lower than 19 is considered too thin. Readings above 25 indicate a person is getting into an unhealthy weight range.

Height (inches)	Body Weight (pounds)															
58	91	96	100	105	110	115	119	124	129	134	138	143	148	153	158	162	167
59	94	99	104	109	114	119	124	128	133	138	143	148	153	158	163	168	173
60	97	102	107	112	118	123	128	133	138	143	148	153	158	163	168	174	179
61	100	106	111	116	122	127	132	137	143	148	153	158	164	169	174	180	185
62	104	109	115	120	126	131	136	142	147	153	158	164	169	175	180	186	191
63	107	113	118	124	130	135	141	146	152	158	163	169	175	180	186	191	197
64	110	116	122	128	134	140	145	151	157	163	169	174	180	186	192	197	204
65	114	120	126	132	138	144	150	156	162	168	174	180	186	192	198	204	210
66	118	124	130	136	142	148	155	161	167	173	179	186	192	198	204	210	216
67	121	127	134	140	146	153	159	166	172	178	185	191	198	204	211	217	223
68	125	131	138	144	151	158	164	171	177	184	190	197	203	210	216	223	230
69	128	135	142	149	155	162	169	176	182	189	196	203	209	216	223	230	236
70	132	139	146	153	160	167	174	181	188	195	202	209	216	222	229	236	243
71	136	143	150	157	165	172	179	186	193	200	208	215	222	229	236	243	250
72	140	147	154	162	169	177	184	191	199	206	213	221	228	235	242	250	258
73	144	151	159	166	174	182	189	197	204	212	219	227	235	242	250	257	265
74	148	155	163	171	179	186	194	202	210	218	225	233	241	249	256	264	272
75	152	160	168	176	184	192	200	208	216	224	232	240	248	256	264	272	279
76	156	164	172	180	189	197	205	213	221	230	238	246	254	263	271	279	287
BMI	19	20	21	22	23	24	25	26	27	28	29	30	31	32	33	34	35

Recommended Pregnancy Weight Gains (based on BMI)

Pre-pregnancy BMI	Recommended Weight Gain
Obese, >29	15+ pounds (6+ kg)
High, 26–29	15–25 pounds (7–11.5 kg)
Normal, 19.8–26	25–35 pounds (11.5–16 kg)
Low, <19.8	28–40 pounds (12.5–18 kg)

(Source: Institute of Medicine of the National Academy of Sciences (IOM))

encouraged to gain twenty-eight to forty pounds, while women who are already overweight are encouraged to gain between fifteen and twenty-five pounds. It's important to note that low weight gain can result in a low-birth-weight baby (less than five and a half pounds) and can increase the incidence of health and developmental problems. So, if you suffer from an eating disorder, *you must get help immediately;* the safety and health of your child depend on it.

On a week-by-week basis, the recommended weight gain during pregnancy is approximately three and a half pounds in the first twelve weeks, followed by a pound per week for the remaining weeks. Again, you mustn't diet in pregnancy, but to help you stay in control of your weight gain you can make healthier food choices and exercise more. Eating less but more frequently, staying away from high-calorie and high-fat foods, and drinking lots of water can also help you keep your gains in the healthy zone.

Calories and Serving Size—the Critical Elements

With the billion-dollar diet and exercise industry working around the clock to churn out the newest "discovery" in weight control, you'd think the key to weight control was truly a mystery. With the rare exception of people who have medical disorders causing them to be overweight, the bottom line in weight gain or loss is simply this: calorie consumption versus calorie expenditure. To lose one pound of fat, you need to burn 3,500 calories. Likewise, to gain one pound of fat you must eat 3,500 calories more than you've burned. It's as simple as that. While the types of food you eat can play a small role in whether you gain or lose, ultimately calorie consumption is the deciding factor. Now, you don't need to count calories in your pregnancy, nor do you need to be thinking about how to lose weight. But it's important to know that any excess weight you gain is gained this way.

The best way to keep your calorie consumption in a healthy range in pregnancy is to keep an eye on serving sizes. I think most North Americans would be surprised by just what nutritionists consider a proper serving size. For instance, did you know that the large bagels found at most coffee shops and bagel stores count as *six* servings of bready carbohydrates while the small, chewy ones count as two? The Food Guide Pyramid created by the United States Department of Agriculture (USDA) suggests people eat five to twelve servings of grain products in a given day. The twelve servings are intended for large, active men, and the five servings for small, less active women. The American College of Obstetrics and Gynecology (ACOG) recommends pregnant women eat at least four servings from this category of food, but eating one of these bagels already puts you two servings above the recommended minimum. Therefore, it's probably a good idea to choose less dense, more nutritious foods to ensure you get lots of variety in your daily diet. Here are some other examples of serving sizes:

- **Meat:** a cooked portion about the size of a deck of cards, a can of tuna, two eggs
- **Dairy:** one cup, a finger-sized piece of cheese
- **Grain Products:** one slice of regular bread, $1/2$ cup cooked pasta
- **Fruit:** one banana, one apple
- **Vegetables:** one cup of broccoli

What to Eat
While the USDA Food Guide Pyramid remains a good guide for healthy eating for pregnant women, the ACOG recommends pregnant women alter the pyramid minimum servings slightly. Instead of two to three milk and milk-product servings, pregnant women need

Food Guide Pyramid for Pregnant Women

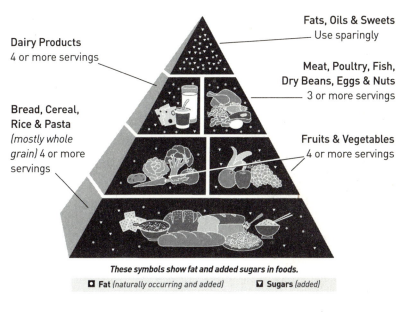

(Adapted from the Food Guide Pyramid created by the United States Department of Agriculture to reflect the ACOG guidelines for pregnancy nutrition.)

four. They also need to boost their meat servings up to three or more, instead of the usual two to three. It's also recommended that pregnant women get at least four servings of fruits and vegetables and four servings of whole-grain or enriched bread or cereal each day. Meanwhile, the USDA says most pregnant women will need about 2,200 calories each day or more. Again, this is a 100- to 300-calorie increase over the recommended prepregnancy caloric intake. Beyond the numbers, however, the key is to stay active, eat healthily, and let your appetite guide your food intake.

Healthier Choices

With cravings, nausea, and hormones sometimes making you just want to head for the cookie jar, you might consider having some healthy substitutions for some of your favorite indulgences in the house. Making just a few substitutions at the grocery store can make a world of difference to your daily calories, fat content count and the overall wholesomeness of your diet. You may want to pay attention to what you are craving, however, as it may indicate something lacking in your diet.

☑ Healthier Choices

	Sample Choices	Quantity	Calories	Fat
☐	Butter	1 tsp (5 ml)	36	4 g
☑	Non-hydrogenated margarine	1 tsp (5 ml)	12.5	1.8 g
☐	2% milk	1 cup (250 ml)	128	5 g
☑	Skim milk	1 cup (250 ml)	90	trace
☐	Ice cream	½ cup (125 ml)	142	8 g
☑	Yogurt, plain	½ cup (125 ml)	79	2 g
☐	Cheddar cheese	1.5 oz (45 g)	181	15 g
☑	Low-fat cheddar slices	1 slice	51	2.9 g
☐	Sour cream	1 tbsp (15 ml)	23	3 g
☑	No-fat sour cream	1 tbsp (15 ml)	11	.2 g
☐	Mayonnaise	1 tbsp (15 ml)	100	11 g
☑	Low-fat mayonnaise	1 tbsp (15 ml)	50	5.1 g

☐	Salad dressing, French	1 tbsp (15 ml)	64	6 g
☑	Fat-free salad dressing, Italian	1 tbsp (15 ml)	15	0 g
☐	Chicken, fried	5 oz (140 g)	364	18 g
☑	Chicken breast, skinless and roasted	3 oz (90 g)	148	3 g
☐	Pork spareribs	2.5 oz (70 g)	235	18 g
☑	Lean ham slices	3 oz (90 g)	130	5 g
☐	Hamburger patty, regular broiled	3 oz (90 g)	260	19 g
☑	Tuna, canned in water*	3 oz (90 g)	143	1 g
☐	Microwave popcorn, 1 bag	8 cups (2000 ml)	200	11 g
☑	Popcorn, air popped	1 cup (250 ml)	25	trace
☐	Apple pie	1/6 of pie	404	18 g
☑	Fig bars	2	100	2 g
☐	Doughnut	1	165	8 g
☑	Arrowroot cookies	2	58	2 g
☐	Corn puffed cereal, presweetened	1/2 cup (125 ml)	114	trace
☑	Oatmeal, cooked	1/2 cup (125 ml)	77	1 g

*Note that, due to high mercury content, tuna consumption should be limited to one serving weekly.

☐	White bread	1 slice	76	1 g
☑	Whole-wheat bread, thinly sliced	1 slice	45	1 g
☐	Large white fluffy bagel	1	600	6 g
☑	Small chewy bagel	1	200	2 g
☐	French fries	10	158	8 g
☑	Potato, baked	1	148	trace
☐	Chocolate chip cookies (6 cm diameter)	2	104	5 g
☑	Orange	1	62	trace
☐	Cheesecake (diameter of 23 cm)	1/12 of cake	278	18 g
☑	Fruit cocktail, canned	1/2 cup (125 ml)	60	trace
☐	Creamed corn	1 cup (250 ml)	194	1 g
☑	Broccoli spears	1 cup (250 ml)	48	trace
☐	Soda	1 can	119	0 g
☑	Diet cola	1 can	0	0 g
☐	Grape juice	1 cup (250 ml)	154	0 g
☑	Tomato juice	1 cup (250 ml)	50	0 g

Eating for Baby and You

Pregnancy creates new nutritional requirements, limitations, and challenges. The baby growing inside of you requires all of the essential vitamins and minerals to grow into a healthy, strong child. Your growing baby also needs you to take certain precautions and preventative measures to help avoid nutrient-related defects. Additionally, the chemical and hormonal changes present the mom-to-be with other challenges, such as nausea. Let's take a closer look at these new developments and at the key nutrients working together to help build your baby.

Folic Acid Fundamentals

Folic acid, folic acid, folic acid. It's one of the first things your health practitioner will discuss with you when you announce that you are planning to have a baby or that you are pregnant. Many studies have shown women who get 400 micrograms (.4 milligrams) of folate (also called vitamin B9) daily prior to conception and during early pregnancy reduce the risk that their babies will be born with a serious neural tube defect (a defect involving incomplete coverage of the brain and spinal cord) by up to 70 percent. That is why the U.S. Centers for Disease Control and Prevention (CDC) recommend all women of childbearing years consume about 400 micrograms daily. Ideally you will begin your folic acid regimen at least one month before you conceive. At the very least, start taking folic acid when you know you are pregnant and continue until at least three months into the pregnancy. While folate can be found in green leafy vegetables like kale and spinach, in orange juice, and in enriched grains, most women need a vitamin supplement to ensure they get the right amount. Be sure to talk to your health practitioner about how much folic acid you need.

> **Pregnancy Food Guidelines**
>
> - Abstain from alcohol.
> - Minimize your caffeine intake.
> - Abstain from shark, swordfish, king mackerel, tilefish, and Mediterranean tuna (due to high levels of chemical pollutants).
> - Avoid artificial sweeteners.
> - Don't eat raw or undercooked meat or eggs.

Calcium

As your baby's little bones and teeth grow inside of you, your need for calcium grows too. Calcium is the essential mineral involved in this development. Also, recent studies have shown increased calcium intake in pregnancy can help protect against preeclampsia, a leading cause of premature birth. It's estimated that 90 percent of American women don't get enough calcium. In fact, most get less than half of the recommended daily amount, and most women are calcium deficient by the time they conceive. So if you are one of those women, it's critical that you correct this before your pregnancy or at least once you become pregnant. The National Institutes of Health recommends pregnant women get at least 1,200 mg of calcium each day. Because most prenatal formulas only contain about 200 to 300 mg of calcium, you should check your bottle to make sure you are getting enough. You can also increase your calcium intake by eating more calcium-rich foods, like milk, cheese, yogurt, and broccoli. Talk to your doctor or health practitioner if you are concerned that you are not getting all the calcium you and your baby need.

"Morning" Sickness

Probably the biggest nutritional challenge faced by pregnant women in the first few months of the pregnancy is nausea, or morning sickness as it's sometimes misleadingly called (for most women, it doesn't stop at noon). As much as 70 percent of women suffer from morning sickness in pregnancy. With our bodies producing increased levels of more than thirty hormones, we can feel positively toxic, making it difficult to find something healthy we want to eat or even to keep food down at all. In fact, at one point in the first trimester, our bodies are making more estrogen in one day than they normally make in three years. You may want to eat that grilled chicken and salad because you know it's good for you and great for the baby, but the smell of the meat cooking on the grill has you running for the nearest washroom! Some women are actually so sick in the first fourteen to seventeen weeks (the usual duration of morning sickness) that they lose weight when they should be gaining, sometimes even landing in the hospital. Short of that, prenatal nausea can cause women to want to eat nothing but crackers all day, staying clear of anything with a smell or a taste. And this isn't the healthiest way to eat. But, you have to do what you can, and for most women this means eating what they can stomach until the nausea passes. Meanwhile, there are a few other things you can do to cope, head off the nausea, and eat well:

- Always keep something in your stomach. If all else fails, try dry crackers.
- Eat a few crackers before you get out of bed in the morning.
- Remember to keep hydrated; try some flat ginger ale.
- Snack before bed.
- Avoid greasy foods.
- Avoid noxious or offending odors.
- Try taking vitamin B6, 25 mg (though the 50 mg over-the-counter version is also acceptable), three times a day: before you go to bed at night for A.M. sickness; when you wake up for afternoon sickness; and at 3 P.M. for evening sickness.
- Rinse your mouth with lemon juice or sniff a lemon.
- Try putting Sea Bands™ on your wrists; they press on an acupuncture point on your wrist to lessen nausea. (It worked for me!)
- Get up slowly.

Nutritional Challenges by Trimester

First Trimester

Morning sickness aside, there are a number of nutritional changes and challenges unfolding in our bodies during the first trimester of pregnancy. With all of the hormonal changes, many women start to develop carbohydrate cravings. This can also be caused by low blood sugar, which is the result of not eating regularly or not eating the right kinds of foods. If you are having carb cravings, you may want to take a look at what you are eating and when your are eating it to ensure you are eating a well-balanced diet and not letting yourself get too hungry. It's important to note that, in the first trimester, weight gain is not as critical as it will be in the last two trimesters, so if you are already overweight, now is the time to be careful not to gain more than the recommended amount. In fact, you don't need any more calories in the first trimester than you did before you got pregnant.

Another challenge women face in early pregnancy is fatigue. Some pregnant women experience exhaustion unlike anything they've ever felt before. If you are suffering from exhaustion, it's important to check with your health practitioner to ensure it's not being caused by an iron deficiency (anemia). Also, don't be tempted to use sugar or caffeine to "wake yourself up." These aids will give you only a short-term boost before making it worse later. And, believe it or not, the best cure for exhaustion is exercise. Get outside, get a little air, and move around a bit. It's amazing what a difference exercise can make.

Second Trimester

The second trimester can be the most wonderful period of a pregnancy. The nausea subsides, as does the exhaustion, and you're starting to look and feel beautifully pregnant. Many women actually begin to feel like they have more energy than ever before. Your belly grows big enough to start wearing cute maternity clothes, but it's not big enough yet to give you too many aches and pains. The second trimester is, however, often marked by problems like constipation, hemorrhoids, and diarrhea. While you should always mention changes like this to your health practitioner, eating fiber-rich foods, like whole grains, fruits, and vegetables, and drinking plenty of water often can make a big improvement. The second trimester is also marked by an increase in appetite. This is totally normal as your body begins to need more calories to build your growing baby. This is when you need to begin eating 100 to 300 more calories each day. Again, keep in mind the number of calories you are burning exercising when making your meal plans for the day.

Third Trimester
As the baby nears its birth weight, your uterus crowds your lungs, stomach, and digestive tract, causing a number of challenges. It gets harder to breathe, indigestion and heartburn become common problems, and many women suffer from hemorrhoids. The best way to deal with these digestive challenges is to eat well. Remember, calcium, iron, and potassium are three of the most important nutrients during this time.

The size of the baby also makes it quite difficult for many women to get and stay comfortable at night, which often leads to insomnia and exhaustion due to interrupted sleep. Eating a high-carbohydrate snack before bed can help you to fall asleep. Pressure on the bladder makes most pregnant women urinate frequently, which can also have them running to the bathroom throughout the night. While it's important to stay well hydrated, it's probably a good idea to do most of your water drinking earlier in the day and stop about an hour before going to bed. Keeping your feet up during the day can further reduce your need to get up and urinate at night. When you go through most of your day without periodically elevating your feet, fluid accumulates in your legs, feet, and ankles. Once you put your feet up, this fluid gets taken off, increasing your need to urinate. If you make an effort to get off your feet once or twice a day—especially if your ankles are particularly swollen—you'll be able to evacuate that fluid at a much more convenient hour and avoid more interruptions to your precious night's sleep.

A Closer Look at the Food We Eat

In order to understand why we must eat a balanced diet covering foods from all of the food groups, we must learn exactly why our bodies, and our babies, need these nutrients. The first thing we need to know is that our energy comes from three sources, carbohydrates, fats, and proteins. Additionally, there are a few other nutrients our bodies cannot live without; they include water, vitamins, and minerals. The following section will go over each of these energy sources and nutrients, explaining why we need them, where we can get them, and how they work together.

Carbohydrates

Carbohydrates are our primary source of energy and are therefore critical to all bodily functions, including building our babies. Fruits, vegetables, and grain products all fall into this category and give us calories from sugars and starches. Carbohydrates are converted to blood glucose in the body, then stored in the muscles and liver in the form of glycogen if not used immediately.

Despite all of the negative attention carbohydrates have been getting in recent years (with the popularity of the high-protein, low-carb diets) experts agree that approximately 55 to 65 percent of our total

Critical Nutrients You Need

Nutrient	Trimester		
	First	Second	Third
Folate	Critical to cell reproduction and division and neural development		
Zinc	Deficiencies in early pregnancy linked to preterm delivery		Critical to baby's brain development and helps Mom heal after birth
Manganese	Critical to development of organs		
Potassium	Be sure to replace these stores if you are vomiting often	Critical for transmission of nerve impulses	
Calcium			Helps build baby's bones
Vitamin A (Talk to your doctor about safe vitamin A consumption levels.)	Critical to cell, tissue, and eye development	Aids in baby's bone and tooth structure	Helps in repairing Mom's cells and tissue damaged during delivery
Vitamin B6	Can be used to treat nausea or vomiting (physician supervision recommended)		
Vitamin C		Helps in production of collagen (part of connective tissue that holds skin together), muscles, and blood vessels	Helps with tissue repair after delivery and aids immune system
Vitamin E			Helps in repairing Mom's cells and tissue damaged during delivery
Iron		Needed for increased blood volume and iron storage in baby	
Chromium		Regulates blood sugar; deficiencies can contribute to gestational diabetes	
Omega-3 Fatty Acids			Critical to baby's brain development
Protein	Key to baby's growth	Creates expanded blood volume, helps growth of breast and uterine tissues, and key to baby's growth	

energy each day should come from carbohydrates. While carbohydrates are essential to fueling everything we do in a day, when our carbohydrate intake exceeds our requirements they can be converted into fat and transported to the fat tissue of our bodies. So, it's important to make sure you aren't eating more than you need.

Simple Carbohydrates
Simple carbohydrates come in the form of sugars or fruits and are absorbed quickly into the bloodstream. If simple carbohydrates are consumed in large quantities, you can end up getting a sugar high, followed by a crash of low energy—and you'll be needing all the energy you can get throughout pregnancy and motherhood!

Complex Carbohydrates
Complex carbohydrates are found in foods like bread, cereal, potatoes, pasta, and rice. They are absorbed into the body slowly, thereby providing the body with a slower, steadier form of glucose. As a result, these are the kinds of foods you want to be eating a day or two before a physical challenge like labor and delivery.

Bread, Cereal, Rice, and Pasta
Aside from giving us the fuel to go about our day, these foods rich in complex carbohydrates give us needed fiber and B vitamins. It's a good idea to choose the whole grain and enriched carbohydrates over the highly processed, fluffy white variety.

Fruits and Vegetables
Fruits and vegetables are great sources of carbohydrates (both simple and complex), fiber, vitamins A and C, and potassium. These foods help our bodies to heal, can reduce our risk of developing cancer and high blood pressure, and can help keep us regular. Fruits and

vegetables also contain certain antioxidant nutrients, which are believed to help reduce the risk of cancer and other disease.

Make vegetables in particular your friends. They are full of vitamins, including vitamin C and beta and other carotenes, potassium, and magnesium. They are water-rich and yummy, and there's a lot to choose from, so take your pick. I like to gorge myself on beets, carrots, and cabbage. The darker and the more colorful the vegetable, the more nutrients it has. Vegetables are also low in calories, so basically you can eat them until your heart (or stomach) is content.

Proteins

Protein, the nutrient responsible for building and repairing muscles, is the building block of your body and your baby. Protein is made up of about twenty different types of amino acid. When the body needs repair, for instance after a run, these amino acids provide the necessary raw material. Proteins that contain all of the essential amino acids are known as complete proteins. These include foods like meat, eggs, and milk products. These complete proteins can be high in saturated fats, however, so it's important to eat them in moderation. The other kind of protein is incomplete protein. This includes foods like cereals, legumes, and nuts. Protein should make up about 10 to 15 percent of your daily intake, but try not to exceed the recommended 50 to 100 grams per day. Protein also helps reduce the risk of iron deficiency and anemia. The best choices for protein are fish and poultry because they are low in saturated fat. Excess protein not needed by the body is easily turned to fat, so it's important to make sure you are not eating too much.

Dairy Products

Milk, cheese, yogurt, and the like all provide our bodies and babies with needed calcium, protein, and riboflavin. These nutrients help to maintain strong bones and reduce the risk of osteoporosis while protecting against high blood pressure. However, it is important to choose low-fat varieties of these foods because they tend to be high in saturated fats. Some of the best *nondairy* sources of these nutrients include tofu, spinach, soy products, and sardines.

Meats and Alternatives

While some meats can be rather fatty, eating healthily doesn't require cutting this food group out of your diet. Meats give our bodies and babies needed amino acids, which are critical to building and repairing muscles. This food group also helps us keep our iron levels in a healthy zone. Choosing less fatty varieties of meats can help you keep your fat content to a minimum while still enjoying your favorite meals. Although the occasional steak is no problem, some of the best choices from this food group include tofu and fish. However, do abstain from certain kinds of fish that contain high levels of chemical pollutants, such as mercury, a neurotoxin that can damage the brain and nervous system of your unborn child. The Food and Drug Administration currently warns against shellfish, shark, swordfish, king mackerel, and tilefish, but advisories have been drafted concerning a popular pregnancy favorite of many women—tuna. It is currently thought that, while Mediterranean tuna should be avoided, Atlantic and Pacific tuna can be eaten safely by pregnant women, but not on a daily basis. To be safe, try to restrict your tuna intake to one meal per week.

Fats

"Fat" has become a dirty word. While a healthy diet includes limiting your fat intake, fats actually need to make up about 30 percent of the food you eat each day. Fat, after all, is the energy source used to fuel long-lasting activity, such as labor and delivery, and is essential to proper fetal growth. That doesn't mean you're free to eat whatever fatty foods you wish. There are "bad" fats, or saturated fats, and there are "good" fats, or unsaturated fats. Saturated fats are found in foods like cheese, butter, meat, and poultry. In many cases you will know saturated fats when you see them because they are solid at room temperature, then get runny when they are warmed up. Unsaturated fats are found in plant sources. There are two types of unsaturated fats: monounsaturated, which are found in olive oil, Canola oil, peanut oil, and avocados, and polyunsaturated fats, which are found in salmon, tuna, and sardines. These are all really good for you. Fats are an important component of nutrition not only because they provide needed energy, but also because they make food taste good and make you feel full. They also help in the transportation of fat-soluble vitamins, such as vitamins A, D, E, and K, and provide essential fatty acids. It's a good idea to choose unsaturated vegetable fats, like olive oil or corn oil, and other fat sources, like walnuts.

Water
With up to 75 percent of our body weight made up of water, and the amniotic sac refilling itself every three to four hours, it's clear why keeping our bodies well hydrated is critical in pregnancy. Water carries nutrients to our cells, helps flush away metabolic waste from cells, and helps regulate our body temperature. It also helps keep our skin clear, lubricates our joints, and cushions our organs and body tissues. We lose two liters (two quarts) of fluid naturally each day, so it's important to keep replenishing our body's supply. We all need to drink eight to ten eight-ounce glasses of water each day. But for active women, especially pregnant active women, it's important to top this off by drinking before, during, and after our workouts. Try to drink

2 cups two hours before exercise, 1 to 2 cups ten to fifteen minutes before exercising, $\frac{1}{3}$ to 1 cup at fifteen- to twenty-minute intervals during exercising, and 1 cup ten to fifteen minutes after exercise.

Vitamins and Minerals

Vitamins and minerals are important for the growth and cellular function of both ourselves and our babies. Essential vitamins, like A, B, C, D, E, and K, control the chemical reactions in our bodies and effect on our fuel pathways. We need them to function. Eating a balanced diet with lots of fruits and veggies, and the appropriate portions of meat and dairy products, can help you avoid deficiencies and the need to take supplements. In fact, with the exception of folic acid, it's generally not recommended that pregnant women take a multivitamin unless they have a known deficiency (iron deficiencies are common after the twelfth week of pregnancy). High doses of vitamins A and E have actually been known to cause malformations in a developing baby. As a result, in 1993 the ACOG advised that extra vitamin A (exceeding 5000 IU daily) not be used during pregnancy. So if you decide to take multivitamins during pregnancy, make sure that you are not taking anything containing especially high levels of vitamin A.

Like vitamins, minerals impact our fuel pathways. Key minerals include calcium, iron, potassium, and sodium. We lose a lot of these minerals when we sweat, so it's important to make sure that your mineral levels do not get depleted from exercising or during labor and delivery. You can get light-headed and weak when certain mineral levels, or your electrolytes, get depleted. Drinking sports drinks like Gatorade™ can help you replenish your stores of potassium and sodium. Bananas or salty treats can also help you replenish these stores.

Recommended Multivitamin and Mineral Supplement for Pregnancy

Nutrient	Amount	% of RDA for Pregnancy
Vitamin B6	2 milligrams	91
Folate	300 micrograms	75
Vitamin C	50 milligrams	71
Vitamin D	6 micrograms (200 IU)	50
Iron	30 milligrams	100
Zinc	15 milligrams	100
Copper	2 milligrams	100
Calcium	250 milligrams	21

(Adapted from the ACOG and the Institute of Medicine of The National Academy of Sciences, 1990, "Nutrition During Pregnancy.")

Foods to Avoid

Caffeine and alcohol are two substances pregnant women would be better off staying away from. While studies have shown that women can consume moderate amounts of each, neither is really good for you, and alcohol can even cause problems for the baby. Caffeine is a stimulant that can trigger your flight-or-fight response, making you irritable, and is a diuretic, which will dehydrate you. You actually have to drink a cup of noncaffeinated fluid for every cup of caffeinated fluid you drink just to replace the fluids the caffeine causes you to lose. Considering how much fluids you already have to consume to stay healthy, this is counterproductive. High caffeine consumption in pregnancy has also been linked to low-birth-weight babies.

As for alcohol, drinking substantial amounts of it in pregnancy can lead to very serious defects in the baby, namely Fetal Alcohol Syndrome. Even smaller amounts of alcohol can affect your growing baby. It's said that by the time you feel tipsy from the alcohol you've consumed, your baby has passed out from the intoxication. That's a scary thought.

Salt is another substance that is often restricted in many women's diets. However, the ACOG advises pregnant women not to restrict their salt intakes. To do so, it says, may be harmful to you and the baby. In fact, your body may require more salt than you're used to eating during the first several months of pregnancy, when your blood volume increases and you need the electrolytes to equilibrate. However, if you develop hypertension in your pregnancy, your health practitioner may advise you watch your salt and sodium intake.

Yet another substance to be wary of during pregnancy is sugar. As we all know, sugar can be found in everything from cookies to candy to cola. Any food that is made up primarily of sugar should be consumed in moderation. It is high in calories and will only give you a short, fast boost of energy.

Getting Fueled Up for Baby

Carbo-Loading for the Big Event

In the days leading up to a long-distance endurance race, such as a marathon, athletes eat additional carbohydrates as fuel for the big event. This is called carbo-loading. Carbohydrates are stored as glycogen in our livers and muscles and are the primary source of energy used during physical challenges. By eating two to three additional servings of carbohydrates, like bread or fruit, in the three to four days before a big physical challenge, you can ensure that your glycogen stores are as full as possible. For women coming close to the end of their pregnancy, it's a good idea to try to load up a bit on carbohydrates to guarantee you've got the energy stores needed to make it through what could be many hours of labor. While few women deliver on their due date, many women deliver within a two-week window around their due date, so once you are about a week away from your due date, you might want to consider carbo-loading. If labor comes before you expected it to, and you're just experiencing early labor symptoms, you may want to start eating some high-carbohydrate snacks to help fuel up for the hours ahead. It's important to note that the idea behind carbo-loading is not to gorge yourself. To do so can actually make you feel lethargic and bloated. You simply want to have a few extra servings each day.

Now, our glycogen stores can actually get depleted pretty quickly during hard physical work. Depending on how hard you are working, they can be depleted in as little as an hour. While that won't likely be the case for your delivery, eventually your glycogen stores will get depleted, so it's important that you keep your blood sugar levels up by refueling with more carbohydrates. Once you are in the hospital (or wherever you plan to deliver), they may not allow you to eat, so find out if that's the case and try to eat beforehand if necessary—and *before* you go into active labor, as eating in the later stages of labor increases the risk of aspiration (a very serious cause of maternal morbidity and mortality). An intravenous line (I.V.), if you have one, will generally have dextrose in it, which will keep your blood sugar in a normal range. Another way to keep up your blood sugar, and therefore your energy, is to consume a carbohydrate drink of some kind. Fruit juices are good and so are sports drinks like Gatorade™. Sports drinks are especially helpful because they replace the sodium and potassium you lose through sweating. But if you haven't tried these drinks before, don't try them for the first time during your labor. You wouldn't want to add a queasy stomach to your other concerns during labor!

Keeping Hydrated

Staying hydrated during a physical challenge is even more important than staying fueled up. As discussed earlier, our bodies are primarily made up of water. Water is critical to carrying nutrients to our cells, flushing away waste, and regulating body temperature. When we become dehydrated, we feel sick, get tired, and aren't able to function at our usual level. And when you are in the delivery room facing the toughest physical challenge of your life, you'll definitely want to be on top of your game. So, unless you have an I.V. for fluids, make sure you stay hydrated. Frequent trips to the bathroom may be annoying and difficult during labor, but it's important that you don't get dehydrated. Try to have a bit to drink every fifteen minutes. And remember, if your urine is dark yellow, you are dehydrated and need to drink more.

Prepping for the Long Haul

In those last few days and weeks before your baby arrives, it's natural to be in a cleaning or planning frenzy preparing for the arrival of your little bundle of joy. While stacking diapers and washing diaper shirts are necessary chores, don't forget to plan ahead on the meal-plan front as well. In the first days and weeks after you come home with baby, you'll be so tired and overwhelmed that meal planning and preparation will be the last thing on your mind. But you will still need to eat. In fact, being up

---

Nutrition Tips

- Make healthy trade-offs.
- Don't be fooled by low-fat foods.
- Buy fresh—not packaged—foods.
- Take time to shop wisely.
- Read labels on food packages.
- Eat snacks during the day.
- Cut *down* on foods, don't cut them out.
- Eat your food slowly.
- Start your day with a good breakfast.
- Make more than one meal at a time.
- Think before ordering restaurant food.

every three hours for feedings is not only exhausting, it makes you quite hungry too! It's easy during this time just to pick up the phone and order takeout. However, takeout food is not the most nutritious of choices and can leave you still needing the vital nutrients required to survive new motherhood. So, plan ahead and cook up a bunch of meals that can be frozen and easily reheated after the baby is born. Lasagna, soups, and chili are some good examples of nutritious, easy-to-prepare frozen dinners you can make ahead of time. What you are going to eat after the baby is born may be the farthest thing from your mind while you are still pregnant, but if you plan ahead you will be very glad you did.

7

Getting Mentally Fit for Baby

Like a marathon runner who visualizes the finish line for months in anticipation of the big event, a mother-to-be can think about the coming physical and emotional challenges ahead of time, making plans and preparing herself as best she can. From taking prenatal classes to writing birth plans to learning breathing and focus techniques, she can mentally ready herself for the big day. And by taking parenting classes, setting up networks of support, and visualizing life with baby, she can arm herself emotionally for new motherhood. While physical preparation is critical to being ready for labor, delivery, and new motherhood, preparing mentally and emotionally is one vital step you don't want to overlook.

Getting Set for Labor and Delivery

Prenatal Classes

Education is probably the most important step to mental preparation for labor and delivery, and the best way to learn all you can about what to expect and how to cope is to attend prenatal classes well before your due date. Knowledge, after all, is essential to alleviating fear and stress about childbirth. A 1991 *Family Medicine Magazine* review of literature on social support and its relationship to maternal health showed prenatal classes decrease maternal physical complications during labor and delivery and improve women's physical and mental health postpartum. Doula Sasha Padron, of the Yoga Space studio in Toronto, says education is critical to feeling strong on labor day. "One of the most valuable things a woman can do to help prepare herself is to really build trust, faith, and confidence in her body and herself," she says. "It's a balance and a matter of educating yourself and informing yourself and finding the people that are going to support you. You have to have that trust and faith in your ability to give birth."

So while these classes usually cost some money (usually not more than $100), rest assured that it will be worth the investment. You'll learn much more about your pregnancy, including how to make pregnancy more comfortable and what to expect in the last weeks before you go into labor. Prenatal classes also go into great detail about comfort measures in labor, prelabor signs, timing contractions, when it's time to go to the hospital, and how your labor support person can help. You will learn about complications, interventions, fetal monitoring, the first, second, and third stages of labor, and the medications and other supports available to you. These classes will also touch on postpartum adjustment and some newborn care. Yet, as many women would tell you, what is perhaps the best thing about these classes is that you are free to ask any questions you may have—no matter how silly, serious, or embarrassing they may seem. Chances are, if a concern or question has occurred to you, it has occurred to countless women before you (and been voiced during one of these question-and-answer sessions).

Classes are usually offered either over several weeks as a series of short evening sessions or in more intensive one- or two-day sessions. The hospital or birthing center you plan to use will likely offer some prenatal classes, and your doctor or midwife will also have a list of prenatal classes to choose from. Remember to ask if you need to bring pillows or something to sit on.

Writing a Birth Plan

While some people may think of this practice as going overboard or a bit of new-age phooey, writing a birth plan is actually an excellent way not only to communicate your labor and birth preferences to your childbirth team but to consider just what your preferences are. If you wait until you reach the maternity ward, you probably won't be in any condition to be making big decisions. You, like many women, might come out of your birthing experience feeling as though you were not in control of some of the things you would have liked to have been in control of, which can be very upsetting. This is the reason for the birth plan. It gives you control of your birth environment even when you are in too much pain to speak or consider your choices. By sitting down and going through possible scenarios ahead of time, you can let your birthing team know what course of action you would like them to follow. Here are some examples of things you might want to cover in your birth plan:

- Will you wear your own clothing or a hospital gown?
- Will you want pain medications, and, if so, which kinds?
- Will you want to be mobile throughout your birth?
- Will you want to be helped into a tub or shower for comfort? (See page 212 for more information on hydrotherapy.)

- ☐ What positions would you like to try for labor?
- ☐ Do you want the baby to be placed on your belly right after the birth?
- ☐ If a cesarean section is needed, do you have any special requests?
- ☐ Do you want to avoid an episiotomy if at all possible?

Some birth plans are several pages long, while others are just a few sentences. It's up to you to decide the thoroughness of your birth plan. If there's a lot you want to cover, don't hesitate to add it in. This is your chance to make known your ideas, expectations, and desires. This is your birth: you get to choose.

That said, it's important that you keep an open mind. You don't know what is going to happen once you are in the labor room, and it's a good idea to allow for a wide range of possibilities. For instance, I had no plans whatsoever to have an epidural, but found myself begging for one after seventeen hours of labor. While I had an extensive birth plan written out, stressing how much I didn't want an epidural, I had nothing written down for what I wanted if I did have one. That left me just following along with what my nurse suggested I do. I hadn't thought through the possibilities and therefore had no input prior to the event. Also leave room for unexpected complications, such as birth by cesarean. Go over your birth plan with your doctor, midwife, and nurse once you go into labor to make sure your preferences are clear.

Visualizing the Day

Imagining the day you get to hold your sweet baby in your arms is something most moms-to-be do almost constantly from the time their doctor confirms a baby is on the way. In fact, for many women, it's hard to think about or concentrate on anything else. While you'll naturally be doing this from the start, as your due date draws near it's a good idea to do some focused thinking about the day you deliver. This can help you to prepare on a number of levels, from making sure your hospital travel plans are set to being just a little more ready for the first time you are left alone with your child. This will help you anticipate the "what ifs" that you haven't already thought of and therefore help reduce stress and worry once your are in labor. Take the time to sit down and thoroughly think out different possibilities of how the day could unfold. Keep a pad of paper and a pen nearby and jot down these possibilities and any plans you make to prepare for them. Ask yourself things like:

- Where am I likely to be when I go into labor?
- How am I going to get to the hospital?
- How long will it take me to get there?
- What am I going to need to take with me to the hospital?
- How am I going to contact my birth partner and where is he or she likely to be?
- Do I have to make plans once I go into labor (e.g., find care for other children)?
- How am I going to alert family and friends that I've gone into labor?
- Is the house going to be in the order I want when I return with the baby?

Taking a tour of the hospital or birthing center you plan to deliver in is critical to visualizing the big day and readying yourself mentally for labor, delivery, and new motherhood. You can see the bed you will deliver in, what the bathroom is like, what labor support aids are available to you, where the café is for your partner to get food from, where you will be taken after the baby is born, how to call your nurse should you need her, and where in-patient breastfeeding classes are held. Once you are there, looking around and thinking about your birth, you'll come up with dozens of questions to ask your tour guide, and the answers you receive will help you plan what to bring to the hospital, know what to expect of the birthing environment, and—best of all—reduce the unneeded stress of the unknown. To schedule your tour, call the labor and delivery office and make sure you plan your tour for at least two weeks before your due date. This is one prelabor step you don't want to miss.

Once you've gone over your upcoming big day thoroughly in your mind and taken the appropriate actions, it's a good idea just to set it all aside and try to clear your head. When those first labor pains begin, you want to be calm and relaxed so that you can let go and know that your body is ready to do what it is designed for—give birth to your child.

Hypnosis

When it comes to coping with the pain of childbirth, no comfort measure should be written off as too wacky to try. While hypnotism has its share of cynics who doubt that people can truly be placed in a hypnotic state with the snap of someone's fingers, many women who have used hypnosis in their labor and birth claim that though it didn't erase their pain altogether, it did reduce it significantly. The purported benefits of hypnotism have also been demonstrated in other medical settings, from the dentist's chair to the psychotherapist's couch.

The idea behind hypnotism in childbirth is that the more relaxed the woman is, the less pain she will have. No one can say for sure whether hypnotism will work for you, but if you are anxious to avoid traditional medical interventions in your birth experience, it may be something you'd want to try.

Keep in mind, however, that using hypnotism in childbirth is not something you try for the first time once you are in labor. Quite the contrary, it takes weeks of education and practice to reap the benefits of hypnotism on your big day. First, you must find someone who is well trained in hypnotism, preferably with extensive experience in the birthing room. These people are sometimes called "hypno-doulas." (To find an expert in this area, you can look under "hypnosis" in the phone book. Be sure to interview any potential hypnotherapists before you sign on, however, to make sure they are qualified, are educated, and have a good reputation.) Next, you will need to attend a number of sessions with your hypnotherapist, learning how to use visualizations to lull yourself into a state of self-hypnosis in preparation for labor. While in the hypnotic state, you are not asleep and will be able to come in and out of the trance at will. The hypnotherapist will act only as your guide, helping you to train your mind to experience the pain as only pressure. You will need to practice this daily on your own. You can also learn how to do self-hypnosis on your own with home study courses found on the Internet. But remember, only 90 to 95 percent of population can be hypnotized, so you might be in the 5 to 10 percent who are out of luck.

Breathing

Breathing techniques can help you in labor in a number of ways. Breathing can help you to relax, help to distract you, and help you keep some kind of control over the birthing process. It's important that you start practicing your breathing early on in pregnancy (the earlier, the better!), so that you will be very familiar with the different breathing techniques when you need them. It's also a good idea to make sure your birthing partner is well versed in these techniques

Relaxation Exercises

EXERCISE ONE: SYSTEMIC RELAXATION

Systemic relaxation, or guided relaxation, can help you cope with the pain of labor. This is something you and your birth partner can practice ahead of time in preparation for your birth. The more relaxed your muscles are, the less pain you will feel during contractions, so find yourself a comfortable position sitting or laying down with your arms relaxed at your sides and have your birth partner read the following script to you and guide you as you try to relax your entire body totally.

> "Now focus on your breath. Try to imagine your breath entering your nose, moving down the back of your throat, and into your lungs. Picture your breath as it leaves your body and leaves you feeling totally relaxed. Let yourself blow away your tension.
>
> Now notice the rise and fall of your abdomen as you breathe in and out. Feel the relaxation coming over you like a warm blanket. Allow yourself to just let go.
>
> Clench your right fist as tight as you can, letting yourself feel the tension as you clench tighter still. Hold your hand clenched and notice the tension in your hand and forearm as well. Now let go and allow your hand to relax. Feel how loose your hand is now. Clench your hand again, then relax, taking time to notice the difference between the tension and relaxation. Now clench your left fist. Hold it, then relax. Allow yourself to let go of all the tension in your left hand and arm.
>
> Now bend both arms and clench your biceps. Tense them as hard as you can and allow yourself to feel all of the tension in your arms. Now, straighten and relax your arms. Allow all the tension to drip out of your fingertips.

Move on now to your head. Wrinkle up your forehead, tense up the top of your head as much as you can. Feel the tension as it crosses over your skull. Now tense up your entire face and feel the tension as it swims across your face. Relax all of your facial muscles now and allow your jaw to drop open. Let the tension drip down off your face as you completely relax.

Tense up your shoulders now, pulling your shoulders up to your ears. Hold this pose and visualize all the tension in your shoulders. Now let your shoulders drop as you relax your neck muscles as well.

Now tense up your abdomen, pulling your arms across your chest as you increase the tension across the front of your torso. Now relax as you let all the tension fall back off of your chest and belly, dripping back into the ground.

Tighten your buttocks and thighs now, holding on tight as you allow the tension to take over your lower body. Let it all out now, relaxing your buttocks and thighs.

Now pull your toes up toward your face, feeling the tension take over your lower legs. Hold it, then release back into relaxation.

Feel the heaviness across your entire body and allow all of the muscles to fully relax. If you feel an area is resisting rest, tighten that muscle for a few moments before allowing it to relax again. This will help you to have awareness of this area and therefore be able to fully relax.

You are now totally relaxed, feeling strong, healthy, and rested. You can feel your breath slowly entering your body, filling up your lungs, and carrying away all of your stress and tension as it flows back out into the air around you."

. . .

Relaxation Exercises

EXERCISE TWO: COGNITIVE CONTROL

During each contraction, your birth partner can guide you through this exercise in an attempt to take your mind to another place, away from the pain. You can use the following "escape locale" or choose one that is special to you. It's important that you and your birth partner practice this ahead of time so that you are ready when you need it. Be sure to let your partner know that he or she needs to get you to your happy place as quickly as possible so that you are already there in your mind once the contraction is at its worst.

> Imagine yourself sitting at the top of a grassy hill in the middle of a field. The sun is shining and the sky is filled with wispy, airy white clouds. The air is warm, but a strong, fresh breeze keeps you perfectly cool. As the sun hits the millions of tiny blades of grass all around you, it creates a beautiful green glint that makes the field look like it's filled with diamonds. Off in the distance a yellow dog is running and jumping, chasing after a butterfly. The butterfly is a large, orange and black Monarch butterfly. It seems to dance through the air, up and down, as it stays just ahead of the dog's snapping, happy snout. You enjoy the sound of the dog barking as you take a deep breath and take in all the beauty around you. You lie back on the warm, soft blanket beneath you and feel the heat soak up from the blanket into your back. You close your eyes and enjoy the warmth of the day.

· · ·

too in order to guide you when the time comes. While breathing basics and patterns will be covered here, it's important that you reinforce these techniques with an expert who can properly instruct and prepare you.

Breathing Basics

Breathing in the labor room is composed of three distinct parts:

1) **The Cleansing Breath:** At the start of each contraction, take as deep a breath in and out as you can. This is called a cleansing breath. This helps to prepare you for the contraction and lets your partner know that a contraction is beginning.
2) **The Focal Point:** It's best if you focus on something while you are doing your breathing in labor. You can focus on your partner, your coach's voice, or a picture of a sleeping baby. It's up to you to choose what you focus on, but it can really help distract you from the pain.
3) **Relaxation:** It's important that you are in a comfortable position whenever a contraction begins. Also, try to relax your entire body as you go into the contraction and stay relaxed until it is over.

Breathing Patterns

There are three key breathing patterns that you can begin as soon as you find the pain of the contractions is causing you to hold your breath. Start with the slow-pace breathing pattern and progress to the modified-pace breathing and pant-pant-blow breathing as dictated by your pain level.

Slow-Pace Breathing
- ☐ Take a deep cleansing breath.
- ☐ Inhale through your nose for four counts.
- ☐ Exhale through your mouth for four counts.
- ☐ Finish with a cleansing breath once the contraction ends.

Modified-Pace Breathing
- ☐ Take a deep cleansing breath.
- ☐ Inhale through your nose for two counts.
- ☐ Exhale through your mouth for two counts.
- ☐ Repeat this pattern throughout the contraction.
- ☐ Take a deep cleansing breath when the contraction ends.

Pant-Pant-Blow Breathing
- ☐ Take a deep cleansing breath.
- ☐ Through your mouth, take three or four short, quick breaths in and out.
- ☐ Follow with a long, relaxing breath in and then out.
- ☐ Continue this pattern throughout the contraction.
- ☐ Take a deep cleansing breath at the end of the contraction.

Getting Set for Motherhood

Parenting Classes

On the first night I had my little boy home with me, a day before my milk came in (it takes a few days for this to happen), I remember being up at 3 A.M. in tears as my husband frantically flipped through our baby book trying to figure out why our baby wouldn't stop crying. In my postpartum pain, sleep deprivation, and hysteria, I honestly thought he'd be crying like that forever.

While my husband and I had taken prenatal childbirth classes, and taken careful notes, we had skipped the parenting classes. Having been Auntie to two nephews at that point, I thought I knew all I needed to know about taking care of a baby. Boy was I wrong. There are so many questions you have in those early days of parenthood, so many questions that you can't even imagine having before the child is in your care. Taking parenting classes before the baby comes can give you valuable information on a wide range of topics, including breastfeeding, coping with crying, colic, adjusting to parenthood, baby's growth and development, when it's time to call the doctor, nutrition, diaper rash, car seats, games and toys, and much more. Attending these classes will help arm you with knowledge so that you'll be more in control and less stressed when you face these challenges with your own baby. Often these classes will continue on into the early days of life with baby, or have a postpartum equivalent, which you will no doubt find to be an invaluable resource once the baby has arrived.

Networks of Support

Next to education, support is the most critical component of being emotionally prepared for new parenthood. You can't do it all alone. It's essential that you have access to family and friends who can lend a hand, a shoulder to cry on, or tidbits of advice on the phone. So you might want to take the time before the baby arrives to take stock of who can help out and how and make a list of their phone numbers so you've got them close at hand when you are flustered in the early days with baby. It's probably a good idea to give these people a phone call ahead of time, too, to make sure they will be available and see what help they can provide. Some friends can bring over meals for you, Dad, and baby, some can throw a load of laundry in while they visit, and others may actually volunteer to take shifts with the baby while you get some needed rest.

Friends and family aren't the only people who can help you out in your early days of parenthood. Groups like La Leche League (breastfeeding experts), your local public health facility, and postpartum support groups are all great examples of other places you can look to for help. It's a good idea to have these numbers on hand, too, in case you need them.

Visualizing Life with Baby

When I was pregnant with my son, I remember imagining his sweet little self toddling down the hall from the bathroom to our bedroom. I pictured this adorable soul, standing about two feet tall, smiling up at me. I tried to envision his face and what his hair would look like. I daydreamed about what it would feel like to hold him. I think this is a pretty common occurrence in pregnancy. Feeling that tiny life growing so quickly inside of you often makes it hard to think about anything else but your baby and how your life will be after you give birth. Not only is this natural, but it also helps you to prepare for life as a mother.

As you daydream about your new baby and how he or she will fit into your life, you are making plans and mental preparations for motherhood. Doing this helps you to organize by planning where you'll place diaper buckets and making sure always to have some formula on hand in case you need it. But visualizing life with baby helps you to ease into the role of a mother on a more emotional level, too. Having imagined that sweet baby in your arms so many times, it makes it a little less of a shock when that baby is finally placed in your arms for good.

There's an interesting theory regarding this phenomenon that takes place during pregnancy. According to Daniel N. Stern, M.D., and Nadia Brushweiler-Stern, M.D., authors of *Birth of a Mother: How the Motherhood Experience Changes You Forever*, there are actually three pregnancies going on at the same time. The first is the obvious growth of the baby; the second pregnancy is the formation of the motherhood mindset; the third pregnancy is the formation of the imagined baby. The doctors say in the eighth and ninth month the mother actually starts to push away her imagined baby "as if mentally preparing [her]self for the real thing." Conflict often arises, they say, if the real baby and the imagined baby are too different. These differences make adjusting to motherhood more difficult and can lead to problems like postpartum depression and bonding difficulties. So while it's natural, normal, and quite useful to dream about what your baby will be like, it's important not to idealize your baby and to try to keep an open mind about what motherhood, and your baby, will ultimately be like.

Setting Aside Control
Talking to other first-time parents, you'll realize that one of the biggest mental challenges of new parenthood is letting go of the control you once had over your life. Even if they aren't control freaks, most people are amazed by just how much their lives change, and continue to change as the baby grows ever so quickly. Just when you think you've mastered all that is involved in the current stage, the child grows and starts doing something new, leaving you struggling to learn how to cope yet again. Sleepless nights aside, this was probably the hardest part of new motherhood for me. I was so used to having control over every aspect of my life that I found it very difficult to just let go and go with the flow. For instance, on some unreasonable level, I desperately wanted my son's diaper to stay clean once I had changed him. I wanted that job to stay "done" and would get quite frustrated ten minutes later when he'd poop again (as new-

borns tend to do) and need to be changed. That's the thing with new motherhood: you have to just laugh and set aside the desire to have everything just so. You do not have control over everything. In fact, the harder you try to organize and control things in the early days with baby, the more out of control it all seems.

I also found it very hard to give myself permission just to relax, heal, and bond with my baby. I was in such a hurry to get up and out of bed and rush around doing all of the things I thought a new mother should be doing. While the dishes do pile up, and you do start wearing the same clothes over and over again, it's critical that you take the time in the first days and weeks of new motherhood to unwind, stay in bed, and take care of yourself and your baby. For many women who are used to a hectic, frenetic pace in their lives, this may be very hard. So, it's a good idea to start planning for this ahead of time. Write down your intention to just focus on yourself and the baby and plan for it. While you are packing your bag for the hospital, put a pile of diapers, a bunch of extra nightshirts, and anything else you feel you might need right beside your bed at home. If you plan to give up control and lay down the framework to help it go smoothly, it will be easier for you to take the time to ease yourself slowly into this new crazy world of motherhood.

Your New Life

Many women today think about how they are going to tell their boss they are pregnant almost before they think about how they are going to tell their partners. Career is a big part of many women's lives these days and is therefore a big factor to consider when planning a family. While it's likely that you will have hammered out all of the details of when you will be off work and when you plan to come back, it's a good idea to think about the bigger picture as well:

- ☐ Who will take care of the baby once you return to work?
- ☐ Do you need to alter your work schedule to fit around the new demands of baby?
- ☐ Do you even want to continue to work full time once the baby comes?
- ☐ Can you delay plans for winning that promotion for a while?
- ☐ Is there a job-sharing program at your place of work that will allow you to spend some time at home with baby?
- ☐ Would working from home be an option you'd consider?
- ☐ Would your partner consider going part-time to help care for the baby?

While the answers to most of these questions won't be known until long after the baby is born, it's a good idea to start thinking about how your life will change once you are a mother. Thinking ahead and starting to consider all of your options can help you to be less stressed and make better decisions when the time comes.

8

The Power of Rest

While being active is crucial to arriving at your due date in top form, you've got to rest that baby-carrying body as hard as you've worked it. Rest and sleep are critical to your body's ability to support the growth of your child, keep healthy, and be strong come labor day. Not to mention the fact that the last few months of pregnancy will be the last days you'll have to sleep and rest whenever you want for what will likely be years! According to the National Sleep Foundation (NSF), not getting enough sleep and rest can reduce our productivity, affect our mental health, make us irritable, reduce our concentration, and weaken our immune system. And with so much going on within a pregnant woman's body, with so much energy being expended, it's all the more important that we get enough sleep and rest in pregnancy.

You'll undoubtedly find that your sleep and rest patterns are impacted by your pregnancy, but there are things you can do to encourage restorative rest, such as taking "mini-rests" during the day, doing relaxation and breathing exercises, learning the value of massage in pregnancy, and avoiding stress. With so much planning and preparing to do, it's easy for pregnant women to forget to make time for rest, but sleep and relaxation need to be among your top priorities throughout these nine months.

Sleeping for Two

So, we know it's important to sleep and rest in pregnancy, but for many pregnant women it's easier said than done. In fact, in an NSF poll, 78 percent of pregnant women surveyed reported they had more disturbed sleep while pregnant. The physical symptoms of pregnancy that can negatively affect a woman's ability to sleep include leg cramps, fetus movements, nausea, body aches, heartburn, the need to urinate, and general discomfort. When the mental symptoms that commonly accompany pregnancy, such as depression, anxiety, and worry, are also thrown into the equation, a good night's rest starts to sound like an unattainable dream.

The reasons for a pregnant woman's difficulties with rest are varied and change from trimester to trimester. In the first trimester, higher levels of progesterone tend to increase our feelings of sleepiness. Meanwhile, this is when pregnant women first find that the pressure from their growing uterus on their bladder and the increase in kidney function (caused by an increase in blood volume) is causing them to wake up more often in the night to urinate. Both of these factors have a negative impact on how rested a pregnant woman feels. In the second trimester, the increase in blood volume and kidney function levels off, while progesterone levels remain high, thereby improving sleep. Later, the movement of the baby and a general inability to get comfortable have most women reporting their sleep still isn't as good as it was prepregnancy. In the third trimester, sleep disturbances hit their high point, with leg cramps, sinus congestion, snoring, insomnia, an increased need to urinate, and general discomfort causing most pregnant women to wake periodically in the night. According to the NSF, one study reported

97 percent of women wake in the night on a regular basis during the third trimester.

Getting the Rest and Sleep You Need
The NSF recommends that everyone get at least seven to nine hours of sleep each night. In addition, it would be ideal if you could also have a one-hour nap in the afternoon. For many pregnant women, particularly in the first trimester, it's hard to go through the day without having a nap at some point. And this is a good thing. Let your body tell you how much sleep you need and don't hesitate to go with it. Your body is working hard and needs all the rest it can get. With that said, there is such a thing as overdoing it, even with sleep in late pregnancy. As a general rule, aim for the amount of sleep each night that you would have considered a good night prior to pregnancy.

Sleeping Tips

Here are some other tips for getting a good night's sleep:
- Cut back on the amount of fluids you drink before bed.
- Exercise regularly.
- If you have swelling in your feet and ankles, put your feet up while lying on your side when awake to help move that fluid out via the kidneys.
- To prevent heartburn, avoid spicy, acidic foods and elevate your head on a pillow.
- Avoid caffeine and alcohol.
- Work on improving your sleep environment. Make it dark, cool, and quiet, with comfortable pillows and sheets.
- Establish regular bedtimes and wake times.
- Avoid high-sugar or salty foods.

Now, getting that quality sleep, as we've discussed earlier, can be difficult. But by following a few easy pointers, you can improve your ability to fall asleep and *stay* asleep. First, it's important that you try to sleep on your left side while pregnant. You can't, for obvious reasons, lie on your front, and lying on your back is not recommended by the middle of the second trimester. Although lying on your right side is acceptable, lying on your left side allows for optimal blood flow to the baby and to your uterus and kidneys. Also, try placing pillows under your neck and right leg, or between your legs, to maximize comfort. Many pregnant women also find it helpful to hold a pillow in their arms, above their bellies, while they try to sleep. There are actually long pillows especially made for pregnant women that can make sleeping more comfortable.

THE SLEEPING POSITON

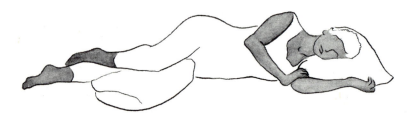

Put Your Feet Up

Sleeping, naps, and relaxation exercises aside, there is a lot of restorative value in just taking it easy whenever you can throughout the day. Whether it's lying down on the couch with your feet up while talking on the phone (instead of standing or sitting at the kitchen table) or making the decision to stay in on a Friday night, there are a lot of opportunities for you to kick back and fit in some basic relaxation. We have worked hard at our jobs and at keeping our bodies and babies healthy, and we deserve to rest whenever possible.

It's a good idea to work more rest into your plans for the coming months as well, as taking it easy during the last weeks of pregnancy is critical to being ready for the big day. You may resist the idea of slowing down; it may be a real challenge for you, especially if you're typically a very active person. But those precious moments of rest give us a chance to reflect, ask questions, and face our fears.

I remember my doctor warning me about a long road trip I planned to take with my husband when I was seven months pregnant. She told me how her pregnancy trip to New York City had had her panting and reeling at the length of a city block, looking for a bench. I didn't listen, however, and found myself moving at a snail's pace through the streets of Halifax. While I could still run a 5K at that point, I wasn't conditioned for all the energy expenditure involved in traveling. (It's more than you'd think.) I'm not advising you to stay at home and have no fun in your last months of baby-free time, but do try to take it easy whenever you can. You want to be rested come labor day—trust me.

Avoiding Stress

There truly is a mind-body connection. In the short term, stress can cause sleeplessness, fatigue, anxiety, poor eating, overeating, backaches, and headaches. Over a longer period of time, it can lead to potentially serious health problems like high blood pressure, heart disease, and lowered immunity. There may even be a link between stress and preterm labor. A growing amount of evidence suggests that stress can generally have a negative health impact on your growing baby. Specifically, research has linked chronic and acute stress in pregnancy to low birth weight and problems with fetal development.

With all of the emotional and physical changes going on in a pregnancy, it's common for pregnant women to suffer from stress to some degree. From the health of the baby to money concerns to the future in general, there's lots to worry about. Some stress over these things can be good, to the extent that it helps us be prepared and get things done that we need to do. But when it builds up to unhealthy levels, it can have a negative impact on our emotional and physical health and be harmful for pregnant women. So, it's important to avoid stress when you can, recognize if you are too stressed out, and do something about it.

Massage
Massage is one of the most wonderful, restorative, and relaxing things you can do for yourself while pregnant. You can do it to yourself, have your partner massage you, or go to a professional. While most of us can't afford to pay for a masseur to massage us daily, it would be ideal if you could massage yourself or have you partner massage you every day. Massage helps relieve stress and tension, eases pregnancy discomforts, and can improve circulation of blood to the baby. Pregnant women who are massaged also have less leg

Stress-Coping Tips

Here are some ways you can help alleviate stress and avoid it altogether:
- Identify what's bothering you and try to resolve it.
- Eat well and regularly.
- Get lots of sleep and rest.
- Tell people not to burden you with unnecessary worries.
- Stay clear of alcohol, caffeine, and cigarettes.
- Exercise regularly.
- Seek out a good support network.
- Meditate.
- Take a prenatal yoga class.

and back pain and lower levels of stress hormones. Belly massage with oils can help your abdominal skin to stretch (although it's debatable whether any cream or massage can fend off stretch marks), and the baby will enjoy it, too. Some of the other benefits of prenatal massage include:

- promotes relaxation
- provides physical nurturing
- reduces tension and aches
- relieves spasms and cramps
- alleviates stress on joints
- combats tension, headaches, and fatigue
- eliminates natural waste products of the body

It's very important, however, that you ask your health practitioner if it is okay that you receive a massage in pregnancy. While massage is usually safe in most low-risk, healthy pregnancies, there are a number of situations in which it might not be safe for a pregnant woman to be massaged. These conditions include, but are not limited to:

- threat of miscarriage
- premature labor
- preeclampsia (unless under a physician's orders and supervision)

When it comes to massage, going the professional route is ideal. You can choose from a variety of different massage types, from light or deep Swedish massage to acupressure and reflexology. The best part of a professional massage is that you can be massaged nonstop for almost as long as you want, from thirty minutes up to an hour

Relax!

Calm Your Mind

The following self-relaxation exercise can be used to help you sleep or just relax during the day. Begin by assuming the proper side-lying pregnancy position on your left side, with pillows comfortably supporting your head and neck and with a pillow between your knees. Make sure you have chosen a quiet place, with dimmed light, and perhaps a nice breeze. Taking nice, big, slow breaths in through your nose and out through your mouth, close your eyes and go through the following relaxing images in your mind:

> I am taking this time to relax, to calm down and to reconnect with myself, my body, and my baby. I am relaxing my head, my neck, and my face. I am letting all of the stress flow out of my head and neck and letting it flow down into the ground. My shoulders are relaxing and all of the tension is dripping down out of them into the earth beneath me. My arms are relaxing now; the muscles are letting go of all the stress and anxiety of my day and I can feel them getting heavier and relaxing. My hands are releasing my tension; my hands are dropping down deep into the ground. My chest is slowly filling with air and with every exhale I am releasing more tension and feeling more relaxed. My torso is expanding; it is open and growing with my baby. I can feel my child growing and moving inside of me. My body is a place of nourishment and love for my child. My hips are open and relaxed. With each breath they are sinking deeper, down deep into the ground. My legs are weightless; they are drained of any tension and stress. My feet relax and dip deep down into the ground below. I am at peace. I am relaxed.

Breathe Deep

When you haven't got time to do yoga or sit down for a full relaxation session, you can center yourself and calm down quickly with a breathing exercise. You need only a few minutes to make a big difference. Once you are done, you can go on with your day feeling refreshed and more relaxed. Good breathing also helps improve blood circulation and oxygenation and is very helpful to both mom and baby in the delivery room. The following breathing exercise can be done anywhere, at any time, and can help you to keep calm and centered in the beginning stages of labor.

1) Sit down with your shoulders relaxed, head in a neutral position, and hands in your lap.
2) Close your eyes and take a nice deep breath through your nostrils and blow out through your mouth.
3) Now, take your right or left hand and gently place your pointer finger and thumb over your nostrils (don't press on both nostrils at once).
4) Press gently on one nostril as you slowly inhale to a count of five through the other nostril. Allow your chest to rise and fill with air slowly.
5) Now, gently press on both nostrils and hold your breath for three counts.
6) Then release the other nostril and release the air out of that nostril to a count of five.
7) Then inhale to a count of five through that nostril. Repeat.

. . .

and a half. (One hour is probably all you'll need.) Getting a professional massage is something you may want to plan to do once a month throughout your pregnancy, and perhaps more regularly as the due date approaches. Athletes often get a massage about a week before the big event.

To massage yourself, you can start with your temples during a bath (not too warm) and follow it up with an overall body massage with cream or oil after you dry off. Get your fingers good and greased up and massage as aggressively or gently as you wish, making sure always to massage in the direction of your heart (this helps circulate blood back to the heart). You may also want to enlist the aid of a rolling pin in your self-massages. Rolling the pin up the back of your legs, up the fronts of your thighs, and along your back can be very exhilarating and relaxing.

If you are going to lasso your partner into massaging you (it's the least he can do, don't you think?!), be sure he keeps his fingers well oiled and follows your instructions on where, how, and how hard to massage. Remember, place yourself in the side-lying position, on your left side, with pillows strategically positioned for support. Get him to start at the top of your head, massaging your scalp, face, and neck, then work his way down. While relaxing you, these massages also give you and your partner a chance to reconnect, giving your partner the chance to show you attention, support, and love.

That Nesting Instinct

In the weeks and days before a baby is born, a mother-to-be is often bitten by a nesting bug that has her polishing wood floors, feverishly shopping for those last few baby items, and cooking up loads of postpartum meals to freeze. Veteran moms often use this event as a superstitious marker indicating that the baby is just days away from his or her arrival. Whether there is an actual biological or chemical change occurring in the mother's body is uncertain, but it makes sense that pregnant women would get a surge of energy before the big event, helping them prepare. That said, don't overdo it. These are your last days to relax before your body and mind are put to the test by labor, birth, the care of a newborn, and recovery from delivery. Make the most of these days. Take care of yourself and take time for yourself. If possible, take a week or two off of work or get a babysitter to watch your other children during the time period directly before your due date. Resting up for labor, delivery, and new motherhood is critical to your body's ability to cope and quickly recover.

9

Countdown to the Big Day

At last, you're in the home stretch. That sweet angel you've been dreaming about for months will be in your arms soon. As they make their way into the final weeks of pregnancy, many women find themselves feeling not only excited, but also anxious, bored, and even frustrated that they can't simply press fast-forward and have that day arrive right away. Perhaps this is because they have spent so much time thinking and preparing and planning that they just want to get on with it. It's in these final weeks, however, that much of the real preparation for baby can finally begin.

While you have been gathering bottles and diapers and blankets, you may have hesitated to start organizing your nursery and actually putting those baby socks in the baby's drawer. There is still plenty to do to prepare for baby and a lot to do to prepare *you* physically and mentally for the arrival of your child. Many first-time moms also don't fully appreciate the fact that these last weeks and days before baby will be the last they'll have to do so many things they will not be able to do for a long time. This is a time to tie up loose ends, a time to make those final preparations, and a time to be savored.

Two Months before Baby

- ☐ Take childbirth classes.
- ☐ Write your birth plan and make copies for your doctor or midwife and hospital staff.
- ☐ Drink lots of water and eat well.
- ☐ Start interviewing pediatricians for the baby.
- ☐ Consider getting nude or clothed pregnancy photos taken (you'll be glad you did).
- ☐ Get your birth partner thinking about his or her physical preparedness for labor, delivery, and the postpartum period. Cardio workouts will help stamina while upper body weight-lifting will prepare the upper body and back for carrying baby.
- ☐ Keep tabs on the baby by counting its movements in an hour. You should be able to count ten movements in two hours. If your baby seems inactive, drink juice to get it moving. If that doesn't work, call your health practitioner.

Six Weeks before Baby

- ☐ Start doing daily perineum massage.
- ☐ Check for inverted nipples and take appropriate action (see Chapter Five).
- ☐ Have a heart-to-heart talk with your husband or partner about expectations and baby care sharing to avoid arguments after the birth.
- ☐ Register for postpartum parenting classes and a postpartum moms' support group.
- ☐ Set up baby's sleeping, diapering, and play areas in the house.

One Month before Baby

- ☐ Pack your bag for the hospital.
- ☐ Practice your route to hospital.
- ☐ Make sure you are eating well and drinking lots of water.
- ☐ Start preparing and freezing meals for after baby is born.
- ☐ Go out for a fancy dinner with your husband or partner.
- ☐ Plan a girls' night out with your friends (no alcohol!).
- ☐ Enjoy a night to yourself, doing whatever you like to do (and won't be able to with a baby in tow).

Signs of Labor

- Leaking or gushing of fluids from vagina (your amniotic sac breaking)
- Expulsion of mucus plug from your cervix (a thick, sometimes blood-tinged clump of goo)
- Aching lower back
- Menstrual cramp sensations
- Tightening of abdomen

Three Weeks before Baby

- ☐ Add pelvic bulging to your Kegel exercise routine.
- ☐ Go shopping for nursing bras.
- ☐ Tie up loose ends with baby plans. (Put sheets on the crib mattress, wash the baby clothes, buy diapers, etc.)
- ☐ Start watching for signs of labor.
- ☐ Eat well, rest, and sleep.
- ☐ Sleep in whenever you can.
- ☐ Nap whenever you can.
- ☐ Continue to exercise and stretch.

Two Weeks before Baby

- ☐ Start carbo-loading (see Chapter Six for details on eating more carbohydrates).
- ☐ Begin breast massage (see Chapter Five for details on breast care).
- ☐ Rest as much as possible.
- ☐ Try to take this time off from work.

What to Have Ready for Baby

Clothing
- 4–6 diaper shirts
- 6 stretchy jumpers with feet
- 4–6 pant/top outfits
- 4 bibs
- 1 hat
- 4–6 receiving blankets
- 6 pairs of socks
- 2 sweaters or jackets

Extra Clothes for Winter Babies
- 2 blanket sleepers
- 1 snowsuit
- 1 warm hat
- 1 stroller blanket

Nursery Accessories
- 2 crib blankets
- 4 crib sheets
- 1 waterproof crib pad
- 2 hooded bath towels
- 6 washcloths
- Infant tub
- Brush and comb
- Nail clippers
- Nasal aspirator
- Ear thermometer
- Diaper pail
- 40+ disposable diapers or three dozen cloth diapers with four diaper covers

Toiletries
- Baby wash soap
- Baby shampoo
- Diaper rash ointment
- Infant Tylenol
- Rubbing alcohol (for belly-button care)
- Cotton balls

- ☐ Watch for signs of labor.
- ☐ Stop weight training.
- ☐ Continue with cardio workouts and stretching.
- ☐ Continue with squats and pelvic tilts.
- ☐ Eat light, frequent meals that are high in carbohydrates.
- ☐ Eat some protein, too, but stay away from fatty or spicy foods that could be hard to digest or upset your stomach (you don't want to worry about this if you go into labor).

One Week before Baby
- ☐ Watch for signs of labor.
- ☐ Get a massage.
- ☐ Continue to exercise and stretch.
- ☐ Sleep in.
- ☐ Take naps.

The Final Days before Baby
- ☐ Watch for signs of labor.
- ☐ Make sure you know where your partner is.
- ☐ Continue to exercise and stretch.
- ☐ Wait for baby!

Packing Your Hospital Bag
- Insurance information, identification, and hospital forms
- All of your labor aids (music, massage oil, comfort items, etc. See Chapter Twelve for labor supports)
- Camera/videotape recorder
- Gatorade™ and water bottles for fuel in labor
- Nightgown, robe, nursing bra, panties, slippers
- Toiletries
- List of phone numbers of friends and family
- Snacks for after delivery
- Loose-fitting, comfortable clothes to wear home (remember your belly will still be quite large)
- An outfit and hat the baby can wear home (keep the weather in mind)

10

The Big Day

Just as a marathon runner goes to the starting line the day before the race, takes a tour of the route, and tries to visualize how the run will unfold, you, as an expectant mother, need to learn as much about the upcoming birth as you can to prepare for The Big Event. When you have some idea of what's going to happen, you can *be* better prepared and you can *feel* better prepared. While every woman and every labor are different, there are many elements of labor and delivery that are the same across the board. By taking a closer look at the three stages of labor and how labor and delivery typically progress, we'll learn to recognize the signs of approaching labor, how to tell when true labor has started, how to cope with labor pains at home, and how to time contractions. We will also talk about how long labor can last, the truth about the pain, what to eat and drink in labor, fetal monitoring during labor, and inducing labor. Now let's learn more about "Labor Day."

Signs of Approaching Labor
Before real labor begins, there are often some signs that labor is approaching. While these indicators can't tell you exactly when true

labor will begin, they can be helpful by alerting you to the fact that is likely to begin soon. The following are signs of approaching labor. If you are experiencing any of these symptoms, monitor them and keep your health practitioner informed.

Lightening: Approximately two weeks before your labor begins, your baby will "drop" down into your pelvis, something known as "lightening." (For moms who are having their second or subsequent children, this dropping may not occur until they are actually in labor.) Once this happens, there is less pressure on the diaphragm and the mom-to-be feels as though it is easier to breathe. One downside of this, however, is the fact that the baby is now placing greater pressure in the groin area and on the bladder, so you may notice that you have to urinate more often as the bladder's filling capacity decreases.

Prelabor: Irregular and often painless contractions of the uterus are known as Braxton Hicks contractions. Many women start to experience these in later pregnancy. While they are not an indication of the onset of true labor, and do not therefore actually dilate the cervix, they do soften the cervix in preparation for labor.

Loss of mucus plug: The mucus plug acts as a seal to the uterus during pregnancy. Once this goopy, gloppy plug comes away, tiny blood vessels in the cervix break, causing a small amount of bleeding. This is not a reason to go to the hospital, but it is a sign that labor is near; once this has happened, labor is likely to begin within a week to a few days to several hours.

Diarrhea: Diarrhea is one of the side effects of the change in the hormones responsible for contractions. As labor draws closer, you may find you are having loose, watery stools regularly. If you feel well besides this, it's likely that it is just a result of the impending labor.

Nausea and vomiting: Some mothers feel the need to vomit as the baby's head presses down upon her cervix. This is normal, but tell your health practitioner about it. Also, make sure you stay well hydrated. A diluted sports drink mixture may help keep you hydrated and fueled if you are having trouble keeping anything else down.

Nesting: Many women get a surge of energy that makes them want to start cleaning the floors and getting the house ready for the baby. This is normal and natural, but it's important that the mom-to-be remembers to take it easy and stays close to home.

True Labor or False Labor?

They say "you'll know" when true labor has begun. That was what my doctor told me a couple of weeks before I went into labor. Still, when I started to get contractions, I found myself wondering if it was the real thing. Initially I was getting mild contractions that were pretty irregular. They'd stop when I got up and walked around and never really hurt that badly. I, of course, wanted to believe the real thing had begun, so I sat up late the night before I officially went into labor reading a book in the position that seemed to keep the contractions coming! The next day, however, it was clear the real thing had begun. The contractions were three to five minutes apart and were getting progressively more painful. Walking didn't stop them; in fact, I'd have to stop walking and stop talking when they did come. And those are some of the typical characteristics of true labor pains. The chart on the following page highlights the differences between true labor and false labor. You can use this chart to assess your own contractions when they begin. Be sure to keep your health practitioner informed of your progress.

Coping at Home

For a number of reasons, you will likely want to stay at home for as long as you can, if it's medically advisable to do so. Unlike the

True Labor vs. False Labor	
True Labor	**False Labor**
Regular contractions	Irregular contractions
Contractions getting longer and stronger	Contractions do not get stronger
Contractions get closer together	Contractions do not get closer together
Contractions get stronger with time	Contractions lessen with time
Cervix opens	Cervix doesn't change

hospital waiting area and delivery room, your home is comfortable, familiar, and free of any restrictions. While there are various reasons why you may need to go straight to the hospital (things your health practitioner will share with you), the early stages of labor will be more manageable if you are in your own space.

Depending on how strong your contractions are, you may want to take a nap or even try to go to sleep for the night (both of which I would strongly advise if you can manage it—especially if your contractions are mild). Or you could curl up with your birth partner, family, or friends and try to watch a DVD or just gab and get excited about the imminent arrival of your baby. You should be timing your contractions once they become strong and regular (see the following pages for details on timing contractions) and keeping your health practitioner informed of your labor symptoms. As your labor progresses, you can start using some of the comfort positions and measures that can help to ease the pain of the contractions (these are outlined in Chapters Thirteen and Fourteen) as needed. In the meantime, have your bags packed and be ready to head to the hospital at any time. Your health practitioner will advise you on when it's time to go to the hospital.

Timing Contractions

While he or she should be well versed in the many ways to give you comfort during labor, your birth partner may be at a bit of a loss initially for what to do to help you when your contractions first begin. Timing your contractions is an excellent job for your labor coach to assume once you are in labor. The laboring mother isn't likely to be in any shape to time them herself past a certain point and shouldn't have to be bothered with an added job.

The time between each contraction is vital information your health practitioner will need to help determine when it's time to head for the hospital. While it may seem like an easy enough thing to do, it's not as easy as you might think—and it's important that your birth partner learn how to do it correctly.

Sample Contraction Timing Chart

Count	Start Time	End Time	Duration	Frequency
1	10:30:20	10:31:15	55 seconds	
2	10:35:20	10:36:05	45 seconds	5 minutes
3	10:40:15	10:41:15	60 seconds	4 min, 55 sec

1) First, you need a watch or a clock with a second hand. You are timing from the start of the contraction to the end of the contraction. That is the *duration* of the contraction.
2) Next, you need to note the amount of time between each contraction, or the *frequency* of the contractions. That time is determined by the difference between the start time of the first contraction and the start time of the second contraction. You can begin timing either when Mom tells you a contraction has begun or when you feel her belly harden under your hand (something some people have trouble feeling).

3) Using a contraction timing chart (see the sample chart on page 187), record the start time of the contraction, the end time, the duration, and frequency for reference.
4) Time four to five contractions in a row, then stop for a while. You can start to time them again when the mother-to-be thinks they have changed (e.g., are getting closer together or stronger). Once you are at the hospital, this job will likely be continued with a fetal monitor.

The Three Stages of Labor

Labor is divided into three stages: The first begins with contractions and ends when the cervix becomes fully dilated. The second starts once the cervix is fully dilated and you can start pushing and ends with the delivery of your baby. The third stage lasts from the delivery of your baby until the delivery of the placenta or "afterbirth."

First Stage: Cervical Effacement and Dilation

Before a woman having her first baby goes into labor, her cervix (neck of the uterus) is usually about two centimeters long and is basically closed. Once contractions begin in the first stage of labor, the contractions pull the cervix up into the bottom part of the uterus, essentially shortening the cervix—a process called "effacement." Eventually, and slowly, the cervix also opens up (dilates) to ten centimeters.

Contractions begin at the top of the uterus and radiate down through the body of the uterus. Where the mom-to-be generally feels them, though, is just above her pubic bone in the front or in her lower back. As the contractions slowly increase in strength, frequency, and duration, the cervix effaces and dilates. Usually the cervix effaces before it dilates, though with a second baby or subsequent babies, both can occur at the same time.

The main phases of the first stage are the "early" (or "latent") phase and the "active" phase. Many people also refer to a "transition" phase, which literally occurs when women are transitioning from the early to the active phase.

Early Phase (Cervix generally 0–3 cm dilated)
How it feels: You will likely feel regular or irregular contractions that are mild to somewhat painful.
What to do: During the early phase, stay home, try to relax, and time your contractions. Have something light to eat and make sure your bag is packed.

Transition Phase (Cervix generally around 4 cm dilated)
How it feels: Contractions become very intense now. You may feel nauseous, become shaky, have chills, and feel the urge to push (but you shouldn't).
What to do: This is when you switch to the pant-pant-blow breathing method (see Chapter Seven).

Active Phase (Cervix generally 2–7 cm dilated)
How it feels: Most women find the contractions quite painful during the active phase of labor.
What to do: Once you have moved on to the active phase of labor (when you can no longer speak comfortably during a contraction), it will probably be time to head for the hospital. (Consult your health practitioner on when he or she wants you to head for the hospital.) Start to use your beginning-stage breathing techniques to help ease the contractions.

Note: How quickly you progress through these phases of the first stage of labor depends upon the shape and size of your pelvis, whether you've had a child before, the size and position of your baby, and the intensity of your contractions.

Second Stage: Full Dilation to Baby's Delivery

The second stage of labor begins once the cervix is fully dilated to ten centimeters. This is when the mother begins pushing. The baby's head will cause her to feel intense rectal pressure at this stage, similar to the need to have a bowel movement. This stage can be managed by the use of an epidural, which can take away the mother's urge to push. (Ultimately, this normal urge to push will come back if you let the epidural wear off.) Fetal monitors or a labor nurse can tell a mother with an epidural when she's having a contraction and can therefore push. This second stage can last as long as one or two hours with a first baby, and ends once the baby has been delivered.

Third Stage: Delivery of the Placenta

You may think that the birth is over once the baby has arrived. But actually the mother still has one more thing to deliver: the placenta. That's the organ that's been nourishing and removing wastes from the baby for nine months. After birth, the uterus continues to contract and shrinks with every contraction. As this occurs, the placenta starts to peel away from the sides of the uterus. The placenta is usually delivered within the first thirty minutes after delivery, but can take up to forty-five minutes to finally come away.

The First Hour After Delivery

During the first hour after the baby has been born, the uterus continues to contract to control bleeding from the site inside the uterus where the placenta was implanted. The blood vessels bleed less as they are squeezed by the contractions. If this is not happening effectively, there is increased bleeding. Intravenous oxytocin (a synthetic form of a hormone that causes contractions) is often given after delivery to help this. Breastfeeding your baby also causes your body to produce oxytocin, which helps the uterus contract. You will feel cramps as the uterus contracts.

How Long Will Labor Last?

The average length of labor for a first-time mother is sixteen hours from start of contractions to delivery of the baby. However, that doesn't mean *your* labor will be that long. Some women deliver within a few hours of their first contraction, while others have been known to be in labor for days. Every woman is different. The possibility that your labor could go on for quite some time is a big part of why it's so important to shape up for labor and delivery and new motherhood. Early labor is the longest stage, usually lasting eight to ten hours, or longer for first babies. This stage is characterized by mild contractions that are usually five to ten minutes apart. The active labor stage usually lasts six to eight hours with first babies and three to five hours with subsequent births, with contractions one minute long and about two to five minutes apart. The transition phase is usually quite short and has contractions about one minute apart that last up to ninety seconds. The pushing stage can last anywhere from fifteen minutes to two hours. Placenta delivery, meanwhile, happens about fifteen minutes to one hour after birth.

The Truth about the Pain

It can be hard to find honest descriptions of the true degree of pain involved in labor. When I was pregnant, I was lucky enough to read Naomi Wolf's book *Misconceptions: Truth, Lies, and the Unexpected on the Journey to Motherhood*. In it, Wolf does a great job of painting a picture of just what level of pain is involved. Wolf points out that in the nineteenth century, doctors described labor pain as one of the most agonizing experiences known to medicine, "more painful than the suffering of soldiers on Civil War battlefields." One woman in her book also describes the pain as torture and worried she'd be haunted by it forever. Part of the reason why descriptions like this are so hard to find, I believe, is that many mothers think good mothers don't complain about things like this. However, the truth is that pregnant women, and women who plan to have children, have the right to know just what they are getting into. It's important to note, meanwhile, that the degree of pain felt by women in labor can vary quite a bit. I've heard of women who simply winced during each contraction and didn't need any medical interventions. In my case, I was completely unprepared for the level of pain. Having run three marathons at that point, I thought I knew pain and thought I could handle it well. The pain involved in running a marathon doesn't even come close to the pain involved in labor. Eventually the pain was more than I could handle and I began to shiver and panic.

In the labor and delivery class I took before my son's birth, the teacher handed out Ziploc™ bags of ice. She told us to squeeze them in the palm of our hands for one minute to simulate the pain of a contraction. At the time I thought this probably wasn't a very good indicator of how much pain was involved, but in retrospect I think it's a good way of getting a sense of the beginning stages of a contraction. By about fifty seconds in, you will probably really want to open your hand and drop the bag. By sixty seconds, it gets pretty intense. I would say my contractions started off that bad, then continued on for another thirty seconds or so, getting worse and worse before easing off. If you attempt this, try to hold the bag for longer than a minute and remember that with a real contraction, you can't just let go of the bag to make it stop.

The amount of pain you feel during each contraction can be affected by fear or anxiety, size and position of baby, previous birth experiences, and your positioning and ability to move around. But most important, the pain is dependent upon the strength and frequency of contractions. The stronger, closer together contractions may hurt more but they get the job done faster. You should also know that your body makes natural pain relievers called endorphins, which, fortunately, will make you feel relaxed and sleepy between contractions.

Eating and Drinking in Labor

There is a bit of controversy over what, if anything, you should be eating and drinking during labor. On the one hand, some medical professionals prefer you to stick with limited amounts of clear fluids in labor because of fear that vomiting could cause breathing problems or that the food could be aspirated if you end up needing to be put under anesthesia. Meanwhile others insist that studies have shown being allowed to eat and drink as you please during labor results in shorter labors, less need for labor augmentation, less need for medication, and babies with higher APGAR scores (a scoring system used to assess the health of the baby in the few minutes after birth). Discuss this issue with your health practitioner ahead of time and find out what rules, if any, are in place at the hospital where you plan to deliver. Some hospitals actually have special labor diets and can provide you with food and drink they think is appropriate.

In my opinion, it's a good idea to keep hydrated and fueled up during your labor. You may not feel like eating or drinking much, but nibbling on a few crackers can help keep your blood sugar up, while sipping on juice or Gatorade™ can help keep you energized and hydrated. You don't want to get dehydrated or hungry during labor. The last thing you need is to feel light-headed, headachy, and faint while you are facing the toughest physical challenge of your life.

Fetal Monitoring

It's important for the professionals supporting you in your labor and birth to know how the baby is coping with the contractions. The following are the different ways to keep tabs on the baby during labor and delivery.

Intermittent external monitoring. This form of monitoring, also known as auscultation, involves your labor nurse using a stethoscope or handheld ultrasound device to check on the baby's heart rate every fifteen minutes or so. One benefit of this kind of monitoring is that it allows you to stay mobile, which may help contractions progress.

External electronic monitoring. This form of monitoring involves measuring the baby's heart rate and the contractions of the uterus through two electronic devices that are secured to your belly with an elastic belt. Both readings are printed out on paper or shown on a computer screen while the fetal heart rate can be seen on a digital display. External electronic monitoring can be done continuously or intermittently to check on the baby.

Internal electronic monitoring. This type of monitoring involves attaching a small electrode to the scalp of the baby's head. The electrode is a tiny curly wire that hooks into the baby's scalp, rarely causing even minimal damage. This is the most accurate way of keeping tabs on the baby; however, it makes you completely immobile and is therefore usually reserved for situations where there is concern about the baby.

Induction of Labor

There are a number of scenarios in which your health practitioner may want to induce labor. If you go past forty weeks and labor still hasn't begun, or if labor begins, then stalls, or if you've got a medical condition that makes continuing to carry the baby problematic, they may want to induce you. Other reasons for inducing labor include the baby not growing well, having low levels of amniotic fluid, membranes rupturing with no signs of labor, a medical problem with the baby, or even for convenience. The ways to induce labor outlined below can get things moving, but aren't without risks. Inducing labor can cause fetal distress and increase the need for a cesarean section (C-section). Many moms-to-be without complications try natural methods of inducing labor once they have passed their due dates, such as activity, intercourse, and taking castor oil. Here are a few other ways to get things started:

Topical prostaglandin. Prostaglandin is a hormone that is naturally produced by the body and can induce labor. A gel containing this hormone can be applied in the vagina or cervix to help the cervix soften and dilate.

Rupturing membranes. If you are close to labor, or if labor is proceeding slowly, your health practioner may break your amniotic sac. Usually he or she will use a long, plastic stick with a hook on the end, called an amniohook, to break the sac gently. (You won't feel the hook—there are no nerves in the membranes!)

Intravenous Pitocin. Pitocin is a synthetic form of the hormone oxytocin (which stimulates labor) and can be given to the mother via an intravenous drip. However, this drug needs to be carefully controlled to create a normal labor pattern.

Stripping the membranes. This involves your health practitioner running a gloved finger along the membranes connecting the amniotic sac to the uterus. This causes the release of your own prostaglandin, which gets labor moving.

Nipple stimulation. This is another method you can do yourself at home, but only with the permission and instruction of your health practitioner. It causes you to release some oxytocin, stimulating contractions. To do this properly, roll your nipple between your fingers for fifteen minutes on each side throughout day.

Once labor has begun, either on its own or after being induced, your baby is on its way — and there's no turning back now!

11

Positions for Labor and Delivery

Once upon a time—and not so very long ago—women went through labor flat on their backs and moved only when it was time to put their feet up in stirrups and push. The idea behind the immobilization of women during labor and delivery is rooted in the twentieth-century medicalization of birth. While ideas like this made labor and birth more convenient and tidy for the doctors and nurses involved, they slowed labor, increased the pain of the contractions, and left the laboring mother feeling helpless and not in control. (Lying on your back can also decrease blood flow to the placenta.)

By going farther back into history and looking at birthing customs around the world, we see practices that are much more conducive to a faster, more comfortable birth that gives the mother some control. As mentioned earlier, in at least one African tribe, women in labor set out for a long, slow run around their village. While this may be the last thing most women in the Western world may want to do once they go into labor, getting up and moving around is the best way to minimize pain and help labor progress. By moving and changing positions often in labor, you can enlist the aid of gravity in bringing the baby down into the birth canal, reduce the discomfort of the contractions, distract yourself from the pain, and enhance your sense of control. Certain positions for labor and delivery can also change the shape and size of your pelvis, allowing your baby's head to move down and rotate in the second stage of labor. Movement helps to ensure the baby gets a continuous supply of oxygen as well. Getting up and moving around can also reduce the length of labor. According to a 1986 study, the progress from 3- to 10-centimeter dilation is 50 percent shorter in women who change positions frequently during labor.

In the following pages, you'll find some of the best positions for labor and delivery. Many of these positions are very effective and beneficial, but tiring; that's why you must get your muscles in shape for this big day. When deciding which ones will work best for you, talk to your doctor and your partner (some of these will require another person's support). It would also help to focus your workouts on the "suggested exercises" listed for the positions that interest you. Also, keep in mind that because holding any position can become tiring, and because movement can help bring the baby down into the pelvis, you should change positions as often as you can.

First-Stage Labor: Coping with Contractions

WALKING

Keep upright and on the move. Don't go too far from home or the hospital and lean on your birth partner when needed for support during contractions.

Advantages: Walking in labor gives gravity the opportunity to help bring the baby down into the birth canal, can make contractions less painful, can help backache, may speed labor, and helps to align the baby with the angle of the pelvis.

Disadvantages: Doing a lot of walking in labor can become tiring. This position often can't be used if the mother has high blood pressure and won't be possible if continuous fetal monitoring is needed. If you want to walk in the first stages of labor, be sure that you also take the opportunity to rest.

Suggested Exercises: Walking, running, cycling, swimming, squats, lunges

STANDING

Keep upright in labor as much as possible. For support, you can lean on your partner, a wall, the edge of your bed, whatever you find comfortable.

Advantages: Like walking, standing during labor allows gravity to work to bring the baby down into the birth canal, can make contractions less painful, can help backache, may speed labor, and aligns the baby with the angle of the pelvis. Standing can also help create the urge to push (in the second stage of labor).

Disadvantages: Standing, too, can become tiring after a while. Remember to lean on your partner and other supports to conserve energy and sit down or lie down and rest if you feel the need. Standing too long causes stasis in the leg veins and can increase swelling in the lower legs, ankles, and feet.

Suggested Exercises: Walking, running, cycling, swimming, squats, lunges

SITTING

You can sit on a birthing ball (see Chapter Twelve for details), your birthing bed, the floor, wherever you feel comfortable.

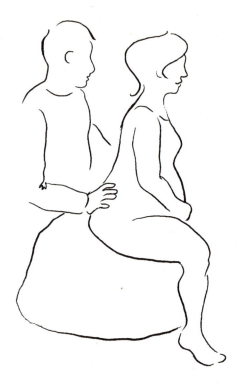

Advantages: Sitting upright allows gravity to bring the baby down into the birth canal while allowing you to get some rest. Sitting cross-legged can also help to open your pelvic outlet.

Disadvantages: While it may be less exhausting than walking or standing, sitting can be tiring and can become uncomfortable if you do it for too long. Also, sitting for a long time, like standing, can cause stasis in the leg veins and increase swelling in the lower legs, ankles, and feet. Moms with high blood pressure may not be able to use this position.

Suggested Exercises: Squats, Chair Abdominal Work, Incline Crunch, Rubber-Band Row, Shoulder-Blade Squeeze, sitting upright with shoulders back

HANDS AND KNEES

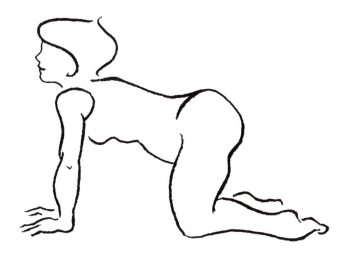

Get down on your hands and knees on a comfortable surface (an exercise mat is great for this). You can also spread your knees and lower your buttocks down toward your feet as a variation of this position. Arching your back occasionally, while on all fours, can also help release tension in your back.

Advantages: This position can help relieve back pain caused by contractions and may rotate babies that are not in the ideal position for birth. This position also allows for vaginal exams during labor.

Disadvantages: This position can get quite tiring after some time. This is part of why it's important to have strong arms and legs going into labor and delivery.

Suggested Exercises: Arm Extensions, Lateral Raises, Baby Hugs, Incline Crunch, lunges, practicing this position

SEMI-SITTING

With pillows propping you up or sitting up against a bed at a 45-degree angle, spread your legs and bend your knees.

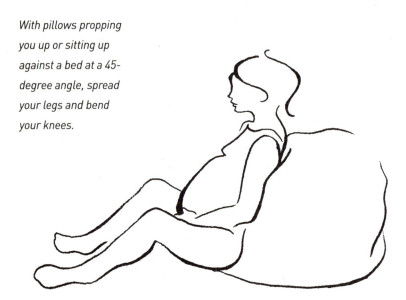

Advantages: This position can work with gravity to bring the baby down into the birth canal and allows you to get some rest. Semi-sitting can also be very comfortable and allows for continuous fetal monitoring. Vaginal exams are also very easy in this position.

Disadvantages: Some women find this position increases back pain. Semi-sitting can also put some stress on the perineum.

Suggested Exercises: Squats, Chair Abdominal Work, Incline Crunch, Baby Hugs, Rubber-Band Row, Shoulder-Blade Squeeze, practicing this position

SIDE-LYING

Using pillows under your head, neck, and leg for support, lie on your left side, and bend your right knee up over the pillow. You can do this on a bed or on a soft surface or mat on the floor.

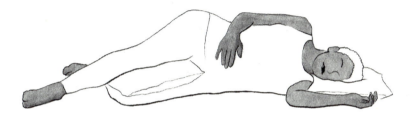

Advantages: This position can be quite comfortable in labor, can lower your blood pressure, and is an ideal resting position. Side-lying can also allow for ideal oxygenation for the baby and is useful if the mother has an epidural. It also promotes good urine production by mobilizing fluid from the legs and by promoting healthy blood flow in the kidneys.

Disadvantages: This position can cause contractions to last longer and doesn't enlist the aid of gravity. Also, be sure to move your legs around frequently to avoid stasis in the blood of your leg veins.

Suggested Exercises: Flapping Fish Pose, the Butterfly, yoga leg stretch (hamstrings), practicing this position

THE DANGLE

With your partner securely holding you up from under your arms, bend your knees and allow your body to "dangle" down. This can also be done with the birth partner sitting on the birthing bed or on a high counter.

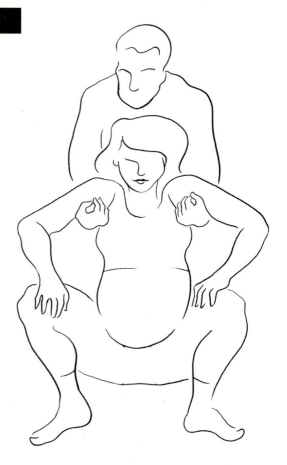

Advantages: This position really helps gravity do its job bringing the baby down into your pelvis. It also allows for no added pressure on your perineum and pelvis.

Disadvantages: Some women may not find this comfortable or may not feel secure in this position.

Suggested Exercises: Squats, lunges, Rubber-Band Row, Biceps Curl, Triceps Extension, Lateral Raises

SLOW-DANCING

Wrap your arms around the neck and shoulders of your birth partner as he wraps his arms around your waist. Lean on him for support as the two of you sway back and forth, breathing together.

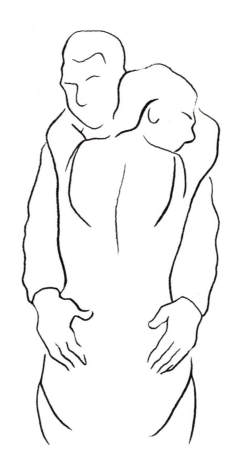

Advantages: This position allows gravity to bring the baby down into the birth canal, can make the contractions less painful, allows the baby to become aligned with the pelvis, and may speed labor. It also allows you to feel emotionally supported by your birth partner.

Disadvantages: This can be tiring after some time and can make fetal monitoring difficult.

Suggested Exercises: Walking, running, cycling, swimming, squats, lunges, Triceps Extension, Lateral Raises, practicing this position

Second Stage Labor: Pushing

While the Semi-sitting and Side-lying positions are also recommended for the second stage of labor, the best position by far at this stage is Squatting.

SQUATTING

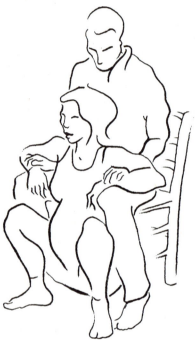

Use a birthing bar (found on many birthing beds in hospitals and used for support during labor and delivery), your partner, or other sturdy objects for support as you squat down on the floor or bed with your feet as flat as possible.

Advantages: Squatting helps to open up your pelvis, giving the baby more room to descend and rotate. Pushing in this position may also reduce the amount of effort you need to put into "bearing down." In this position, your upper body is also helping the baby descend by pressing down on the top of the uterus. Many women find it a natural position for the act of bearing down.

Disadvantages: This can be tiring if you haven't practiced squatting or don't have strong legs and ankles.

Suggested Exercises: Walking, running, cycling, swimming, squats, lunges

12

Natural Supports

Birth is a totally natural process, but nature is not always kind—especially when it comes to the agonies of labor. While we ultimately end up with our arms filled with the most precious gift of all, getting there can be pretty darn painful. Fortunately, modern science has found a number of ways to help women get through the pain of labor and delivery without having to feel the pain to its full extent, and in some cases, to stop them from feeling it at all.

Though these birth backups will be covered in detail in the next chapter, we'll take a quick look at a medical intervention that is used in up to 80 percent of North American births: the epidural. This tiny catheter tube in the spine can numb most of or all of the pain from contractions and birth. While it is popular, and for the most part completely safe, there is a downside to this road to a pain-free birth. Epidurals can cause maternal fever (which can result in your being separated from the baby after birth for testing), increase the need for forceps or vacuum-assisted deliveries, may mean you'll need a catheter to urinate as long as the epidural is in effect, and have been associated with higher cesarean-section rates. There are also a number of rare side effects, including a painful headache if the epidural is not done correctly. For these and other reasons, many women today wish to go the more natural route, or at least hope to. This is part of what this book is all about. Yes, it's important to do all you can to strengthen your body so you feel strong come labor day, but it's especially important if you hope to give birth without medical interventions, such as an epidural.

There are several ways you can improve your chances of "going natural" or at least making yourself more comfortable until you feel you want to use some of the many medical interventions available to ease your pain.

Midwives

Studies have shown using a trained midwife rather than an obstetrician can increase your chance of having an unmedicated delivery by 95 percent. Midwives prefer to deliver babies in a more natural way and work hard to support women in their efforts to give birth without drugs. There is also an argument to be made that using a midwife can improve the quality of prenatal care you receive, if only because of the amount of time she spends with you. Midwives spend an average of forty-five minutes to an hour with patients during prenatal visits while obstetricians average just six minutes. The more attention you receive before and during your labor and delivery, the less anxiety you are likely to have, and therefore the less pain. (Being tense and anxious tightens your muscles and makes you feel more pain.)

While midwives do not always get the respect they deserve, it's important to know that they are fully qualified to take care of you throughout your pregnancy and deliver your baby. They can deliver your child at home, in the hospital, or in a birthing center, where many midwives have their offices. Midwives educate the mom-to-be, help her identify her options, offer emotional support, give medical care, and answer questions. They can also provide all of the prenatal care a doctor can, including checking your blood pressure, monitoring your weight gain, and charting the growth of the baby. When it comes to labor day, many midwives also stay with you for a good portion of the labor, unlike some doctors who may come in only during the pushing stage of labor.

Doulas

Women supporting women through the pain of childbirth is nothing new. But the relatively new idea of hiring a doula is becoming an ever more popular option these days. Doulas are women who provide emotional, physical, and educational support to the expecting parents. Meeting with you a few times before the birth, the doula then comes to you once you are in labor and stays with you the entire time. She will massage you, help you breathe, focus, move around, find comfortable positions, whatever will help. Research has shown the more attention a birthing mother receives during labor, the less pain she feels. Doulas also facilitate communication with the medical staff, explain options to you as they arise, and make an effort to calm the often bewildered dad-to-be. Ultimately, the presence of a doula reduces use of epidurals by 60 percent and cuts C-section rates in half.

Birthing Centers

While most babies in North America are still delivered in hospitals, there is a growing trend toward giving birth in birthing centers. Birthing centers are designed to make your birth experience more comfortable and enjoyable than what it might be in the more clinical setting of a hospital. Usually it's a midwife who will deliver your baby at a birthing center. These centers have a homelike atmosphere, complete with nice beds, decorated rooms, a stocked kitchen, dimmed lights, couches, and carpeting. While medical supplies and backups are on hand, they are hidden to keep the comfortable, relaxed atmosphere. Unlike in many hospitals, you can also have as many friends and family members present for your birth as you want. Meanwhile, the midwife can still monitor baby throughout the labor and delivery and transport both of you quickly to the hospital if required. Midwives are also trained in infant CPR and travel with oxygen. After the birth, the mother and baby usually stay for several hours for observation before being sent home.

Massage

While birth partners *should* be aware of the many things they can do to help ease the pains of labor, sometimes they find themselves flustered and unsure of how to help once the real pain kicks in. One thing they can always do, and that often helps, is massage. They can massage your head, your face, your neck, your arms, your shoulders, your back, your hips, your legs, and virtually any nook and cranny you feel might benefit from some warm, strong hands. It's best if you can take a bath before your massage (see hydrotherapy section on page 212) to help loosen up your muscles and soften the skin. With some kind of good and greasy oil, have your partner use long, firm strokes on your long muscles and knead your shorter muscles.

Guide your birth partner in the massage, indicating where is good and where you'd rather not be massaged. And if it's not helping, tell your partner to stop, or to try massaging another part of your body. You may find massage helps during your contractions, or you may find you can tolerate it only between contractions. Your lower back, the top of your hips (at the back), and the front of your thighs are three areas where laboring women often find massage helps. Now, it's important to tell your birth partner ahead of time to take the initiative once you are in labor because you may not be in any state to be thinking about how a massage might help once you are having strong contractions.

Heat and Cold

Other natural aids that may help to ease your labor pain are hot and cold compresses. An ice-filled baggy, a frozen bag of peas, a cold gel pack, or even a cold, wet cloth can be placed on your lower back or lower abdomen between or during contractions to help numb the pain. You may find these cold compresses can help in other areas of your body as well, or even just placed quickly on your forehead or neck to help you feel refreshed. A heating pad, a rice-filled sock (zapped in the microwave), or a hot water bottle can also be placed on your lower back to ease the pain. Alternating hot and cold compresses is often the best way to ease contraction pain. A hot, moist towel can be placed on your perineum (skin between anus and vagina) to help it relax and stretch. This can also be done with more perineal massage during labor.

Birthing Ball

Squatting is an ideal position for labor and delivery. It opens up your hips and helps the baby descend into the birth canal. It can be hard to squat, however, if you haven't got enough physical strength in your legs and hips. This is one reason why shaping up for labor and delivery is so important. Whether you've practiced squatting and strengthened your legs or not, a birthing ball can help you to sit in a semisquatting position without straining your body. A birthing ball, or exercise ball as it is often called, allows to you spread your legs as much as you want and allow the baby to descend. If you use a birthing ball in your labor, it's critical that you make sure you have a sturdy object, like the side of the bed, to hold onto so you don't fall over. Talk to your doctor to make sure that your delivery room will accommodate a birthing ball. Also, as it's important to keep the surface of your ball clean (you will be sitting on it without underwear on), you may want to cover the ball with a towel before you sit on it, or keep the ball on a clean surface, like an exercise mat. These balls can be found in at least three different sizes, but can usually hold up to three hundred pounds. Try out the birthing ball beforehand to make sure you don't feel too low (go up to the next size if this is the case) and to find out if this is something you think would help you in labor. Birthing balls can cost as little as twenty dollars and can be handy exercise tools to have around after childbirth.

Hydrotherapy

For thousands of years, women have been giving birth in water because of the way it can help ease the pains of labor and delivery. This practice, known as hydrotherapy, is one of the most effective natural aids in labor and delivery, and showers and tubs are now available at most hospitals. The water can help in a number of ways. First, the buoyancy of the water takes stress off of your joints, lessening your overall body discomfort. And warm water, apart from its ability to decrease the transmission of pain signals, is also just plain relaxing. The more relaxed you are, the less tension there is in your muscles, and the less pain you will feel. Jets in a bathtub can provide added massage.

However, because your body gets used to the warmth of the water, the benefits of sitting in a tub or stepping into a shower can diminish over time. So, it's a good idea to get out once it doesn't seem to be working anymore and try again later. After your bath or shower, you can try to sleep. Having a bath or shower is also a good thing to do at the start of your labor, but don't take a bath at home if you think your water has broken, as that could increase your chance of infection. Also, keep in mind that the water you use needs to be *warm, not hot*, and make sure your partner knows not to leave you alone in the tub and to help you ward off dehydration caused by sweating by giving you plenty of fluids.

T.E.N.S. (Transcutaneous Electrical Nerve Stimulation)

In an effort to avoid an epidural (a plan that ultimately underwent some on-the-spot revision), I researched and found a Transcutaneous Electrical Nerve Stimulation (T.E.N.S.) unit. Used by physiotherapists to help stimulate muscles in injured people, these units can be used by laboring women to lessen the pain of the contractions as well. And they really do work. A T.E.N.S. unit is like a tiny, battery-operated Walkman with three wires coming out of it. At the end of two of these wires are four sticky electrode strips which can be placed on your lower back. At the end of the third wire is a little clicking device that you can use to turn the device up and down. Once the unit is on, you feel a tingly, prickly sensation on your skin. When you turn the device up (you have control over its strength) this sensation can be quite strong. Once you begin a contraction, you can click the device up to high, which activates different nerves than those activated by the contractions. This confuses your brain's perception of the pain. You can rent these units from the physiotherapy unit of your hospital or from some pharmacies for about $50 for two weeks. Pick up the unit in good time beforehand to learn how to use it and practice.

Acupressure

I didn't believe so-called "pressure points" on your body could truly have an impact on your pain or your health until I found myself struggling with severe nausea in my first trimester. Desperate for something to help, I ultimately tried Sea Bands™, these little stretchy bands with hard white balls on the inside, which are placed on your wrists. The white balls need to be placed on the exact right spot to help with nausea. Within five minutes of having them on my wrists, I felt normal for the first time in weeks. I was stunned. Whenever I took them off, the nausea would come back, so I started showering with them on! Anyway, I share this story in hopes of convincing you that acupressure, or applying pressure on key points on the body, may help you cope during labor and delivery. Acupressure can help to enhance your body's pain-relief system and deepen relaxation. Have your birth partner begin with gentle pressure and progress to firm pressure with the fingertips, pressing each point for three to five seconds. Points along your neck and head can help with headaches, while points along your spine can help with labor pain or sciatica. When pressing on the points on the back, it's important for your birth partner to apply pressure to the ridges of your muscles on either side of your spine, not directly on your spine. These points on your back are one inch apart along your spine. Pressure points on your feet can also significantly reduce the pain from contractions. Here, have your

CONTRACTION PAIN QUIETERS

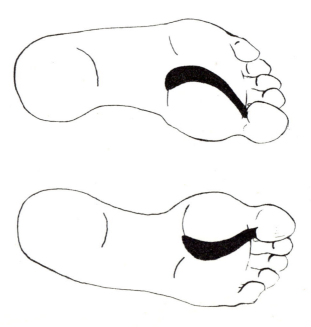

ACUPRESSURE POINTS

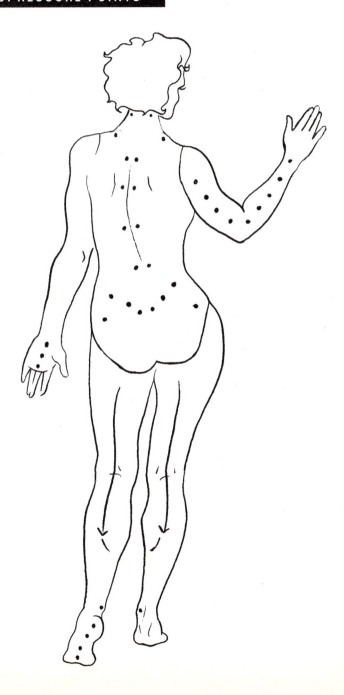

birth partner press four fingers around the ball of your foot and apply intense pressure throughout your contraction.

Music

Whether they are bringing back wonderful, vivid memories, taking us into another world, or even putting us to sleep, songs can have a remarkably strong impact on our mental states. For this reason, music can be a great aid in easing the pain of labor and delivery. If you have a strong, positive association with a song, it can cause you to produce more endorphins, which will help you relax and feel happy. Music can distract you from your pain or relax you, lessening the pain. Listening to music can also help to reinforce constructive activity, like proper breathing. So, if you've got some tunes that you just love, you may want to bring a Walkman and some CDs into the labor room with you. Classical music has been known to have a very relaxing effect on laboring women. Consider bringing a variety of musical options, because you never know what you will be in the mood for once labor begins.

13

Backups You May Need

Whether you plan to have a natural, drug-free birth or hope to take advantage of whatever pain relief is available to you, it's important to remember that things don't always work out as planned. Women who would rather not use drugs or interventions to help them through their births may find themselves needing, and wanting, medical help at some point in their labor or delivery. Alternately, women who planned to use drugs may find things are moving too fast or that they can't have the drugs they wanted for some other reason. Meanwhile, complications can arise that can have you faced with any one of a number of other medical interventions that may be required to keep you and your baby safe. My point here is not to focus on how things might go wrong or not unfold as you expect, but to encourage you to learn all you can about the drug therapies available to you and any medical interventions you could encounter. This chapter will take a closer look at some of these measures so that you can make better choices, both before you go into labor and while in the labor room.

Epidural Block

With 50 to 80 percent of women in United States using it to alleviate their pain in labor, the epidural is by far the most common form of pain management in birth. The epidural block is an injection into the spinal area that numbs the pain-sensing fibers in the spine, essentially numbing you from the waist down. The procedure is almost painless; however, you must remain perfectly still while the needle is being inserted into your spinal area. The needle is then removed, but a small tube is left in your back as a conduit for the medication. That tube is then taped into place on your back. While it does a good job of numbing virtually all labor pain, the epidural is often criticized for making women immobile, slowing labor, temporarily decreasing blood pressure, making it impossible to get to the toilet, decreasing the ability to push, and increasing the need for instrument-assisted birth. Other side effects are also possible, including a rare headache caused when the spinal canal is accidentally pierced by the needle. On the positive side, the epidural does allow you to be alert, hardly affects the baby, and helps you to get some rest before the baby is born. Also, it's possible to get a so-called walking epidural, which allows women to still be able to walk in labor. While some hospitals wait for women to be four centimeters dilated before they will give an epidural, the American College of Obstetrics and Gynecology says women should be given the epidural upon request, once they are deemed to be in active labor.

Narcotics

The second most popular method of pain management in birth is narcotics, given either by injection intramuscularly or intravenously. Two of the most common forms of narcotic used are Demerol and Stadol. Taking about two to four minutes to take effect, these drugs basically "take the edge off" the contractions by acting on your entire nervous system to change your perception of the pain. While narcotics don't restrict your movement or affect your ability to push, they can make you temporarily nauseous, will certainly make you drowsy, and will enter the baby's bloodstream. They may also speed your labor. One of the biggest concerns with this form of pain relief is that the short-term and long-term effects on the baby are not known. What *is* known is that these drugs may slow your newborn's reflexes and breathing if they're not cleared from your system (and the baby's) before delivery. For this reason, narcotics can be given only during labor and are generally stopped before you get to the pushing stage of delivery.

Nitrous Oxide

Known as "giggle gas" to some who've had it in the dentist's chair, nitrous oxide is another relatively common way to lessen pain during labor and delivery. It's important to note that this gas merely reduces the amount of pain your feel and will not eliminate it altogether. The gas is inhaled through a mask that you hold in your hand. You can take breaths in whenever you feel you need it. The effects are almost instantaneous and disappear quickly once the mask is taken away. This method can be used all the way through delivery. Safe, simple, and having no impact on the progress of labor, nitrous oxide is one option worth considering. It can, however, make you nauseous and isn't available at every hospital.

Pudendal Block

While most drugs used to control pain in birth focus primarily on the pain of the contractions, the pudendal block takes aim only at the pain a woman feels in the perineum, vagina, and rectum. The pudendal block is an injection into the pudendal nerve on each side of the vagina, usually to help a woman cope with an episiotomy, instrument-assisted birth, manual removal of the placenta, or repair of a laceration. It also lessens the pain as the baby descends through the birth canal. This local anesthesia is very safe and serious side effects are rare.

Spinal Block

One of the less commonly used methods of controlling pain in birth is the spinal block. An injection into the back, the spinal block numbs all feeling in the mother from the waist down. It is often used in C-sections, and some anesthesia teams may use a combination of an epidural with a spinal. Taking effect more quickly than an epidural block, the spinal block may also be ideal for someone who is close to delivery but wants something in a hurry that may not need to be effective for very long.

Episiotomy

As we've discussed in other sections of this book, the episiotomy (cutting of the area between the vagina and anus) is a controversial procedure. It's debated whether this is a beneficial procedure or whether the mother is better off just tearing naturally on her own. Proponents of the procedure say it is sometimes better if the perineum is cut than if the skin tears naturally and irregularly; certainly, a bad tear can make postpartum recovery more difficult. They also argue that it is medically necessary sometimes to help a distressed baby come out faster. Shortening the time that the baby's head is compressing the mother's pudendal nerve at the very end of labor may in addition lessen the severity and the chance for postpartum urinary incontinence. Critics of the procedure say often episiotomies are done for no reason other than to speed a birth for convenience's sake. The side effects of episiotomies may include difficult recoveries, a greater chance of incontinence, infection, and a risk the incision will lead to further tearing into the rectum. If you don't want to have this procedure done in your birth, talk to your health practitioner. But keep in mind, if the baby is in distress, if it is in a breech position, or if its shoulders are stuck, an episiotomy may be medically necessary.

Forceps/Vacuum

Sometimes when a birth is taking too long it can become dangerous for the baby. In cases like this, your health practitioner may make the decision to help the baby along with forceps or a vacuum. Forceps are a smooth, spoonlike device that fits around the baby's head and allows the doctor to pull the baby out. A vacuum is a suction cup that fits over the head and works with a vacuum pump to hold the head firmly while the doctor pulls the baby out. These instruments are used in about 10 percent of vaginal births. While side effects of their use are rare, a vacuum can sometimes cause temporarily misshapen heads.

Cesarean Section

Sometimes a normal vaginal delivery is just not possible. When this is the case, the baby is delivered surgically through an incision made in the woman's belly. Due to the high risks associated with any major operation, a cesarean section, or C-section, is done only when it's needed to protect the mother and child. One in five babies in the United States is born this way. Situations when a C-section may be required include when there are signs of fetal distress, when the baby won't fit through the birth canal, when labor is failing to progress, and when the umbilical cord is wrapped around the baby's neck or dropped through the birth canal (where it may cut off the baby's oxygen supply). A C-section may also be performed ahead of time for a number of other reasons, including preeclampsia, if the baby is in a breech position (feet or buttocks first), if the placenta is blocking the vagina (placenta previa), or if the placenta is tearing away from uterine wall (placenta abruption). An epidural or spinal block is usually done prior to the C-section, allowing the mother to remain awake. Birth partners are also usually allowed to stay in the room during the delivery. The delivery of the baby takes only about fifteen minutes, but the entire procedure can take about an hour. Meanwhile, it's harder to recover from a C-section than from a vaginal birth. Side effects include incision pain and severe gas pain, and the risk for bleeding is higher than for vaginal delivery. Women usually stay in hospital for at least three to four days after a cesarean delivery. It used to be that women who had delivered by C-section before would have to deliver every child they had via C-section. These days, however, it's possible to have what is called a VBAC, or vaginal birth after cesarean.

14

Recovery

In the first hours and days after the birth of your child—when you actually feel like you've been hit by a Mack truck— you will fully appreciate why it was so important to strengthen your body and mind for this enormous challenge. After the birth of your baby, you will be exhausted and hungry, and will likely have aches from head to toe. Your back will hurt, your vaginal area will be quite sore, your legs may be tired, your arms and shoulders may soon feel the strain of holding the baby, and you may be surprised by the laxity of your abdominal core muscles (from being overstretched during pregnancy). These muscles can provide little support to your back, making simple tasks like sitting up or getting off the bed quite difficult. Meanwhile, you've got a wee child who needs around-the-clock care, including feedings at least every two hours (despite the fact that these feedings may soon enough go for an hour or more at a time!). It's very important to take good care of yourself in the days and weeks after birth, as caring for your baby will put extra demands on an already worn-out, tired body. This chapter will take a look at what to expect and what you can do to make things easier on you — both physically and mentally — as you set about the enormous job of caring for yourself and your new baby.

The First Few Hours

Most women only get a chance to exhale once immediately after their baby is born before that child is handed to them for good. This is what you've been dreaming about for months, but you may be surprised by how quickly it becomes a real physical challenge. If you plan to breastfeed, your health practitioner will probably get you to try nursing almost right away. Breastfeeding takes some time for both you and the baby to get a handle on, so don't get discouraged if things don't work well right away. After the baby's first feeding, don't forget to eat something yummy yourself. You've just completed the biggest "marathon" of your life, so eat something nutritious and hearty. After you are back in your room, it's important to start trying to get some rest. I remember wanting to just sit there looking at my son, and being afraid to close my eyes for fear someone would come in the room and steal him! But when I look back on those first few hours, when he slept so soundly, I wish I had tried to get more sleep. Newborns tend to sleep quite a bit on the first day, but soon the baby will be up regularly. Now is your chance to get that much-needed rest. I can't stress this enough. Perhaps your partner can stay with you and keep an eye on the baby while you nap. You may also want to ask family and friends to hold off on their visits until after you are home.

Vaginal-Birth Recovery

The first time you get out of bed, call your nurse for help. Blood can pool in your legs and you may feel faint and light-headed once you're on your feet. Also, with your core abdominal muscles almost useless at this point, you will need to use your arms to pull yourself up and out of bed. For your first venture out of the birthing bed, a trip to the bathroom is a good goal. Start by bending your knees, rolling onto your back, swinging your legs around the side of the bed, then pulling up using the bars on the side of the bed. Pulling in your perineal area (as you would doing a Kegel) is a good way to lessen pain in that area when getting up in the first postpartum hours and days. Once in the bathroom, try to urinate. You can lessen the sting of urinating by spraying warm water on the area using a water bottle as you go (use this water bottle to clean the area after you urinate as well). It will likely be two to three days before you will have a bowel movement. Your health practitioner may prescribe a stool softener to help this along. About ten to twelve hours after birth, start taking a sitz bath two to four times each day. A sitz bath is a warm-water–filled basin that sits on your toilet and allows you to soak your vaginal area. This helps lessen swelling, soothes the area, and helps to avoid infection.

You will be nursing your baby every two to three hours continuously for several weeks to come. Expect to feel cramps in your uterus as you nurse, caused by your uterus contracting back down to its normal size. Your nipples will probably start to feel quite sore and may even start to crack and bleed from the baby's suckling. You may want to start putting

> **Postpartum Warning Signs**
>
> Call your health practitioner if:
> - Your bleeding becomes bright red and very heavy (you soak a pad in an hour).
> - You pass a blood clot larger than a plum.
> - Your bleeding develops a bad odor.
> - You have a fever of 101 degrees F (38 degrees C) for more than a day.
> - You have difficulty or there is burning when you pass urine.
> - You have increased pain or swelling in your stitches.
> - You have redness, swelling, increased tenderness, or drainage from your abdominal incision (C-section moms).

some Lansinoh ointment on your nipples to help ease the pain. (Lansinoh ointment can be found in most drugstores.) Also, until your milk comes in, let the baby suckle for a few minutes on each side, as often as you like, but not for prolonged periods at one sitting. It's also critical that you support your baby well with pillows or a nursing pillow to minimize strain on your shoulders, back, and arms. Whenever possible, use some sort of support when holding the baby. Overuse injuries in arms, shoulders, and back are very common in new parents. Meanwhile, your health practitioner may give you some painkillers to use as needed in these first few days.

The First Few Days
New moms are notorious for trying to do too much, so sit back, relax, and let someone else do the laundry. In the beginning, although getting up and walking a little bit is fine, try to stay in bed as much as possible. Feeding the baby every two to three hours, and still recuperating from labor and delivery, you may feel too exhausted to do much anyway. But especially in these first few days, make caring for yourself and your baby your top priority, concentrating on nursing, bonding, resting, and keeping yourself well fed and hydrated. Also, don't forget to eat and drink well during these first few days.

Between the second and tenth days after birth, crying, mood instability, and anxiety are seen in 80 percent of new moms. This is normal and natural. While experts aren't entirely sure what causes this, it's presumed that sleep deprivation and the massive hormonal change going on inside our bodies after birth are to blame. If you find yourself feeling this way, try not to feel bad about it and realize it's an experience most new moms have. And do try to get as much sleep as you can; sleep when the baby sleeps!

If you are breastfeeding, the second night with baby can be particularly challenging, as your milk has yet to come in and the baby

Postpartum Depression

While being emotional, overwhelmed, and weepy can be very normal and natural after the birth of a baby, sometimes the so-called Baby Blues don't go away and turn into actual depression. When this happens, it can be very serious. If you fall into any of the categories outlined below, it is critical that you see your doctor and get some help. There is help out there. It's also important to note that 5 percent of new moms develop an autoimmune-related thyroid disorder, which could be causing the problem. So make sure you see your doctor if you have postpartum depressive symptoms, are having trouble losing weight, or seem to be losing weight too quickly.

Signs That You May Need Help
- Feeling that you don't want to be around anyone else
- Feeling hopeless
- Worrying that you might harm your baby intentionally
- Feeling that you don't want to touch or hold your baby
- Feeling confused or disoriented
- Feeling unable to cope

Tips to Keep Sane in the Postpartum Period
- Get as much sleep as you can; when baby sleeps, you sleep!
- Get out of the house at least once a day. Go for a walk with the baby or join a mom and infant support group.
- Go out for a cup of tea or a walk alone as often as you can.
- Cry if you feel like crying and remember—it's all natural.
- Take the phone off the hook.
- Don't worry about how you look; it's pretty hard to keep perfectly groomed with an infant in tow.
- Talk to your partner and friends about any feelings you are having.
- Talk to your doctor if you are upset or concerned about your level of depression.

doesn't seem to feel quite full drinking only your colostrum (the "liquid gold" that comes in before the milk). Remember, though, that a full-term healthy baby has glycogen stores in her liver as well as "brown fat" elsewhere in her body to sustain her for days. Just because babies cry doesn't mean they have low blood sugar, or that they are hungry. Try holding her close, or you can use a pacifier (and still successfully breastfeed!). Also, attending a breastfeeding class in these first days after birth will no doubt be worth the exertion.

In-Bed Exercises

Keeping in line with your need for bed rest, start to do some in-bed exercises the second day after delivery to start strengthening your body again and help meet the physical challenges you are already facing.

- Start with some slow, gentle Kegel exercises. (See Chapter Five.) Do five repetitions, holding for ten seconds, and progress to twenty-five repetitions. Kegels will help you tone your pelvic floor muscles, aid in healing the area by increasing blood flow, and help to prevent incontinence.
- Next you can do some pelvic tilts. Lying on your back, take a deep breath and tilt your pelvis back, bringing your hips toward your ribs. Do twenty pelvic tilts each day. These will help restore your posture and minimize backache.*
- You can begin to strengthen your core abdominal muscles with a simple abdominal contraction exercise. Lying on your back with your knees bent, take a deep breath. On the exhale, pull in your abs. Repeat fifteen to twenty times each day. This exercise will help your core muscles begin to provide some support to your back again.*
- Leg slides can be done while lying in bed and help with your posture and backache. While on your back, bend one

knee and slide your foot along the bed until it comes as close to your buttocks as possible. Be sure to press the small of your back down toward the bed as you do this. Slide the leg back down to the start position and repeat on the other side. Do five slides with each leg.*
- ☐ While sitting up in bed, do some shoulder and neck rolls to encourage blood flow and release tense muscles.
- ☐ Next, it's a good idea to stretch your major muscle groups, either in bed or while standing and holding onto the bed. This will encourage blood flow, make you feel rejuvenated, and start to make you feel like your old self again.

*These exercises require the use of abdominal muscles and are not for women recovering from a cesarean birth.

The First Three Weeks
Well-known Canadian midwife Mary Sharpe advises new moms to spend the first week "in bed," the second week "on the bed," and the third week "around the bed." Most expecting mothers are surprised by the emphasis their midwives, doulas, or doctors place on postpartum rest, but the fact is getting tons of rest needs to be your key focus for the first three weeks. That's not to say that staying in bed that long is easy. On the contrary, it involves some planning and establishing a solid support network.

Get the Rest You Need
- ☐ Have someone stay with you around the clock to help make meals and run errands while you sleep and care for the baby.
- ☐ Don't expect to get a full night's sleep for some time. Consider yourself on the night shift and just try to get all the sleep you can when the baby sleeps throughout the day.

- Have friends and family bring over a meal and run a few errands while they are visiting.
- Resign yourself to having a messy house for a while. The most important job is taking care of yourself and the baby.
- Pace yourself. Try to do just a little more each day.

Your Vagina after Birth

After you give birth, you will continue to feel contractions as your uterus slowly works its way back down to its normal size. These contractions, or cramps, will usually intensify when you are breastfeeding. This is normal. They are also helping clear out the blood within the uterus, which is called "lochia." This process of uterine involution, or return to prepregancy state, will go on for four to six weeks. You will likely have to use a large sanitary pad for the first week or so, and then minipads as the lochia slowly lightens up in both quantity and color. Lochia begins as bright red blood, then turns to rusty brown, then pale pink, then sometimes yellow. Meanwhile, your perineal area may be very sore after the delivery. Use ice packs on your perineum if you find that helps with the discomfort. Spraying warm water on the area and using sitz baths regularly can speed healing and soothe the area as well.

Cesarean Section Recovery

A cesarean section is major surgery. For that reason, it will take even longer for moms who delivered this way to recuperate. C-section moms usually stay in the hospital a few days longer than their vaginal-delivery counterparts and need more help caring for the baby in the early days because of discomfort from the incision and restricted use of their gradually healing abdominal muscles. If you deliver via C-section, your health practitioner will prescribe some pain medication, which you can take as often as you feel you need it. Also remember to pace yourself and not try to do too much too soon. While all new moms need to get as much sleep as they can, rest is even more critical to moms who have had a C-section. In the hospital, your incision will be checked daily by your nurse, and after the bandage comes off you can have a shower. Aside from the pain of the incision, a large amount of gas tends to gather in the bowels after abdominal surgery, possibly leading to considerable gas pain. To help the gas pass, try to avoid carbonated beverages, get out of bed to a chair, do some slow walking, and lie on your left side. Also, eat a high-fiber diet and drink lots of water. Sometime in the first one to five days after giving birth, you can begin doing some deep-breathing exercises, ankle circles, and toe-flexing exercises. Follow your health practitioner's advice on progression of exercise from here. You also need to cough regularly to clear your lungs of any mucus. To get up from your bed, bend your knees, roll onto your side, and use your arms to pull yourself up by holding the bars on your bed. And, by all means, ask for assistance the first few times you get out of bed.

Body Image

Now that your baby is out of your belly and in your arms, you may be surprised at just how big your belly still is! Your uterus stays enlarged for a few days, but the bulk of the belly that remains is caused by lax abdominal core muscles, stretched skin, swelling, and any extra fat you gained in pregnancy. So don't be surprised in the first several days after birth if you still look quite pregnant. This is completely normal. You may be anxious to get your old body back and may find your less-than-svelte postpartum figure frustrating, but remember that the weight will go in time. In fact, most women generally lose fifteen pounds within a few days of delivery, with a total of twenty-four coming off in the first six to eight weeks. Any additional weight you have to lose will come off in time once you get back

> **Average Postpartum Weight Loss by Numbers: Total 17 pounds**
>
> - 7 pounds: newborn
> - 1.5 pounds: placenta (although my sister's was a whopping 5 lbs!)
> - 1.5 pounds: amniotic fluid
> - 7 pounds: body fluids and blood

into your regular fitness routine about six weeks after delivery. It's probably a good idea to wait for at least a week or two before you weigh yourself for the first time. And don't be discouraged if the weight loss isn't as much as you had hoped. You likely still have a lot of excess fluids to shed. Remember: You can get your old figure back with time. I weighed seven pounds less than I did before I got pregnant by six months postpartum. The first few weeks after delivery isn't the time to worry about weight or dieting. Eat well, drink well, and get lots of rest. There will be plenty of time to get back in shape later.

15

Getting Back in the Game

I ran a 26.2-mile marathon seven months after giving birth to my baby boy. A lot of people thought I was crazy, and, in many ways, I now think they were right. But at the time, training for and running that race was critical to my feeling as though I had regained control of my body and life after having a wee passenger at the steering wheel for so long. I loved being pregnant and love being a mom, but pregnancy and early motherhood can make you feel that your body and life are no longer your own.

    Exercise can help you to reclaim your body and life, both physically, by helping to get it back to the way it was prepregnancy, and emotionally, by giving you something to do for yourself. Aerobic exercise in particular can help you to combat the Baby Blues while giving you some much-needed postpartum time alone. Now, I'm certainly not suggesting anyone launch into a marathon-training program right after delivery; most competitive athletes don't even do that. What I do suggest, however, is getting back in the game as soon as you feel you are ready. Many women in the first few weeks after giving birth start to get frustrated with their still-swollen figures and grow quite anxious to begin working out again. But, it's important to pace yourself and learn some postpartum exercise basics. We'll also take a look at how to ramp up your exercise program again, the ins and outs of exercise and breastfeeding, and how to fit it all into your new life as a mom.

When to Start Again

Every woman has to make her own decision about when it is time for her to start regular exercise again after delivery. Experts recommend waiting two to six weeks before starting back. I recommend waiting closer to six weeks or at least until you have had your first postpartum checkup, which usually happens around that time. However, some women have jumped back on the horse immediately after delivery without any problems. A study of a thirty-four-year-old distance runner who started a sixteen-week marathon-training program immediately after giving birth showed that well-trained women can participate in vigorous activity soon after pregnancy. As a competitive athlete, this woman may have had a lot of incentive to get back

---

When It's Not Okay to Exercise Postpartum

Absolute Contraindications
- heavy bleeding
- pain
- breast infection or abscess

Relative Contraindications
- C-section or traumatic vaginal delivery
- breast discomfort
- heavy urine leakage
- heavy pelvic pressure

into such intense training so quickly. Most women don't, and would be wise to take some time to rest, recuperate from both the pregnancy and delivery, and get to know their child. I started to work out two weeks after my delivery and soon found my bleeding intensified. Whenever I stopped, the bleeding would slow down, then I'd try again, and it would start up again. Ultimately I had to wait until seven weeks postpartum before the bleeding finally stopped. I suspect if I had just waited in the first place I may have been able to get back to it sooner. There's something to be said for having a little patience.

The Melpomene Institute has issued the following guidelines for exercising after having a baby:

- If you had an episiotomy, wait until all soreness is gone to start exercising.
- If you're bleeding heavily, or your blood is bright red, wait until bleeding stops.
- Be aware of continuing joint elasticity; it can be deceptive.
- Fatigue is common.
- Drink a lot of water if you are nursing.
- Don't forget to continue to support your breasts.
- Use Kegel exercises for bladder incontinence.
- Watch posture to avoid back pain.
- Make sure you warm up before working out.
- Eat well.

Getting Your Abs Back

The belly. That big, jiggly, sloshing, possibly stretch-marked mound of flesh you used to call your tummy. It's usually Public Enemy Number One for new moms back on the exercise circuit. But before you jump right in there and start doing a hundred ab crunches a day, it's important to check to see if your rectis abdominis has separated. (This test is outlined in Chapter Three.) If the muscles have separated, take special care not to damage them further; follow a modified abdominal workout (outlined below) to begin with.

MODIFIED AB WORKOUT (FOR SEPARATED ABDOMINALS)

1) Lying on the floor with both knees bent, cross your arms over your abdomen with both hands grasping your sides so that they support the abdominal muscles.
2) Tilt your pelvis to flatten the small of your back against the floor.
3) Inhale and, on the exhale, raise your head off of the floor while pulling the muscles together with your hands.
4) Remain in the up position for five seconds before slowly lowering yourself back down.
5) Repeat ten to twenty times.

Note: You can make this exercise progressively more difficult by lifting your shoulders off of the floor as well.

If you have separated abdominals, do only this kind of abdominal exercise in the first six weeks after birth. Once your health practitioner has given you the green light to proceed with regular abdominal exercises, you can move on to the more intense ab exercises that follow this one.

FLAT AB EXERCISE 1: THE PRESS-AND-REACH

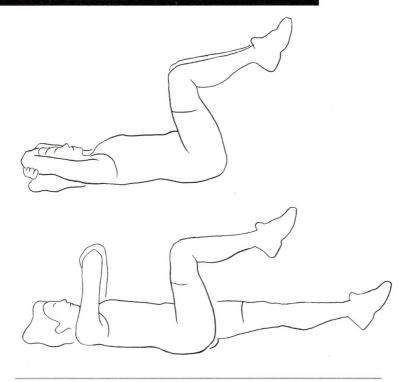

The goal of this exercise is to stabilize your pelvis against the changing resistance of your moving arms and legs.

1) Lying on your back, bend your arms above your head and bring your legs to a 90-degree angle to your body.
2) Holding your elbows and keeping your knees bent, concentrate on keeping your lower back flat as you slowly straighten and extend one leg. At the same time, raise your arms up to a 90-degree angle to your body.
3) Exhale as you extend your leg and inhale as you slowly return to the start position.
4) Repeat with the other leg. Continue for as long as you can manage to keep your back flat.

FLAT AB EXERCISE 2: THE BICYCLE

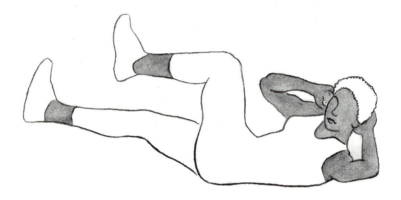

1) Lying flat on the floor with your lower back pressed to the ground, put your hands beside your head.
2) Bring your knees up to about a 45-degree angle and slowly go through a bicycle pedal motion.
3) Bring your left shoulder up toward your right knee, then your right shoulder to your left knee. Remember to exhale and contract your abdominals as you contract up and keep your breathing even and relaxed throughout.

FLAT AB EXERCISE 3: ABDOMINAL CONTRACTIONS

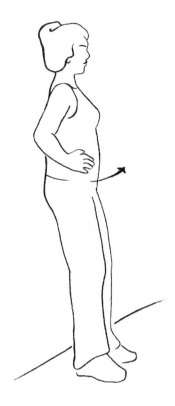

---

1) Lean your back and buttocks up against a wall with your feet about six inches in front, your knees slightly bent, and your hands on your belly.
2) Take a deep breath in and, as you blow out, pull your bellybutton in toward your spine, tilting the bottom of your pelvis forward.
3) Hold for twenty seconds, keeping your abs contracted but breathing throughout.
4) Release and repeat.
5) Do twenty-five reps, five times a day. Work up to one hundred contractions, ten times a day.

Keeping Your Body Strong

As we learned in Chapter Three, early motherhood can put a lot of strain on your muscles from head to toe. As a new mom, you may find your arms, shoulders, and back are pretty sore and tired. While exercising these muscles further with strength training may sound counterintuitive, that's just what you need to do. You've got to keep that body strong to help those body parts meet the challenges they are facing around the clock. The strength-training exercises outlined in Chapter Three can be done in the postpartum period as well. You'll find that the Shoulder-Blade Squeeze, the Rubber-Band Row, and Wrist Curls are particularly helpful in the postpartum period. Remember to do at least two strength-training sessions each week, leaving at least one day of rest in between. And don't forget those muscles people can't see! Keep up those Kegel exercises to help avoid urinary incontinence and other problems often experienced after childbirth.

Keeping Aerobic

You can do all the ab crunches you want and you still won't get rid of that baby belly if you don't incorporate aerobic activity into your fitness regimen. Hopefully, most of your remaining belly is just swelling and loose skin, but some is likely to be unneeded fat as well. The only way to get rid of this is to burn it, and the best way to do that is to get moving aerobically. Once you've been cleared by your health practitioner to start exercising again, you are free to continue with whatever form of aerobic exercise you were doing prepregnancy or start something new. It's up to you to decide what you enjoy and what fits best into your schedule. If you decide to go back to doing the aerobic exercise you were doing before giving birth, be sure to take it slow and only do what feels comfortable at first. Progress slowly, increasing your intensity and duration of exercise by just 15 percent each week. But remember, it's important to participate in aerobic exercise at least three times a week for at least twenty minutes at a time to get any benefit from it. Chapter Two outlines four great beginner workout schedules for swimming, cycling, walking, and running. You can use these charts to help get you back on the road to postpartum recovery and getting that fabulous bod back!

Stretching

We mustn't forget the third prong of a well-rounded fitness regimen—stretching. Having long, supple muscles with a full range of motion is critical to overall health. Stretching out tight, overused muscles also feels wonderful when you've been walking the halls with baby all night! So don't forget to stretch out all of your major muscle groups at least once a day. Also try to work stretching into your warm-up and cool-down routine before and after aerobic exercise. Whenever you feel stressed or have back or shoulder aches, try stretching out those muscles. Over time, these areas will loosen and start to feel like their old selves again. In addition to the new stretch below, use the stretches highlighted in Chapter Four, especially the chest and neck stretches.

The Plow

One of the most relaxing stretches I have found is something called the Plow in yoga. This stretches out your whole back and down the back of your legs. I like to roll from side to side while in this position because it massages all those tense back muscles. It's a great way to give yourself a back massage when there's no one around (or willing) to do it for you! Once I find one of those knots in my upper back, I hold my position, pressing my body on that point. In time, the knot diminishes in size. By the time I'm done, I feel a lot less tense. This position is particularly enjoyable for women whose lower backs have been bent back the other way for nine months.

THE PLOW

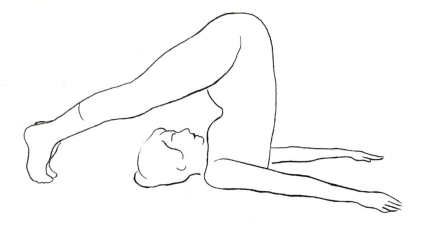

1) Lying on your back, kick your legs up over your head.

2) Hold onto your legs, keeping them straight, and work up to touching your toes to the ground behind your head.

3) Hold as long as you like.

Breastfeeding

There has been a great deal of study into whether exercise affects the quality or quantity of breast milk. One study found that babies did not like the taste of breast milk taken from their mothers after they exercised. Unfortunately, that study was tainted by the fact that those children were breastfed, yet were given the test milk with a bottle. Many breastfed babies show disinterest in bottles. While studies have shown that there is an increased amount of lactic acid, a byproduct of exercise, found in the breast milk of women who exercise, experts have concluded that babies can't tell the difference and that exercise does not affect quality or quantity of milk. However, you may want to consider feeding your baby before you work out. Also be careful to keep your weight in a healthy range and to eat and drink well. Breastfeeding moms need 150 to 500 extra calories each day. It's also interesting to note that experts disagree on whether breastfeeding helps you to lose weight after birth or whether the hormones associated with breastfeeding help you to keep weight on until you wean.

How to Fit It All In

This is the greatest challenge of the postpartum period: Once you have a baby, you wonder how you will ever have enough time to do all you need to do in a day. In the haze of those early days, it seems all you have time for is changing diapers and feeding the baby. You have to rush to find time to shower, you eat on the run, and the dishes never seem to get done. How in the world will you ever find time to work out? Believe it or not, before long you will get better at fitting it all in and can then make exercising a priority. You may feel that working out is a selfish endeavor, and not something you should be taking time away from your baby to do. The truth is, however, that working out will make a happier, healthier you, which makes you a healthier, happier, and better mom to your baby. You owe it to your child to take good care of yourself.

That's all well and good to say, but how do you actually fit it in? Making exercise a priority is the first step. Next, it's important to pick activities that can be done while doing other things. Running or walking with the baby in a jogging stroller, taking a "Mom and Me" yoga class, and doing laps at the pool with baby in a car seat at the end of your lap lane are examples of how you can work out and take care of your child at the same time. My son sleeps, eats Cheerios, plays with his toy bar, and yaks away to himself on our many runs in the park. He seems to love the fresh air, the change of scenery, and the motion of the jogger. You could also run or walk to or from work, lay your baby beside you on the floor while doing your ab work or Pilates routine, or find out about member nurseries in your local fitness club. Where there's a will, there's a way.

Don't Rush It

Some people say it took your body nine months to get into the state it did, so expect it to take nine months for your body to get back to its old self again. While this may be a good time frame to work with, it doesn't have to take this long. If you work really hard at it, you could have your body back in just three or four months. Madonna was performing onstage in low-riding hipster jeans just three months after giving birth to her son, and we've all seen those photo spreads of Sarah Jessica Parker showing off her newly regained washboard abs just a few months after having her boy. While I suspect many a Hollywood siren has simply had her tummy tucked (they apparently just pull down the skin, snip a bunch off, and create a new bellybutton!), if you want a hard belly back, or for the first time, you can have it. That said, I would recommend you give yourself nine months to a year to take it easy and slowly work your way back. It will take your skin and body some time to tighten up and recuperate anyway, so why rush it? Spend the first year of your baby's life bonding and enjoying your child, not fretting over how many inches you have left to take off your waist.

Exercise is terrific for your body and mind, but only if it's not coming at the expense of the things that really matter. And remember: You've crossed the finish line! It's okay to take the time to rest, recover, and really dig into your new job as a mom. You'll need to be both rested *and* strong for this new race you've begun, the Marathon of Motherhood.

Index

A

abdominal contraction exercise, 228, 239
abdominal muscles, 45, 50, 52, 56–60, 92, 228, 235–239
ACOG. *See* American College of Obstetrics and Gynecology
acupressure, 171, 213–216
ADA (American Dietetic Association), 122
aerobic exercises. *See also* cycling; running; swimming; walking: postpartum, 240–241; prenatal, 19–39; safety and, 7–8
"afterbirth." *See* placenta
alcohol, 129, 141, 142, 167, 170, 179
American College of Obstetrics and Gynecology (ACOG): eating guidelines of, 124–125; on epidurals, 218; exercise guidelines of, xxii–xxiii; on salt, 142; on vitamin A, 140
American College of Sports Medicine, xxiv
American Diabetes Association, xviii
American Dietetic Association (ADA), 122
American Journal of Public Health, xxiv
amniohook, 195
amniotic sac, breaking to induce labor, 195
anemia (iron deficiency), 2, 132, 137, 140
ankle circles, 231
ankles, swollen, 134, 167
APGAR score, 193
arm extensions, 64
arms: muscles of, 48–49, 61–68, 86, 87, 92, 240; strength training for, 61–68, 240
aspiration, 143, 193
autoimmune-related thyroid disorder, 227

B

baby: APGAR score and, 193; benefits of exercise and, xxi–xxii, 18; birth weight of. *See* birth weight; birthday of. *See* big day; getting mentally fit for, 147–163;

245

baby: *continued*
   in jogging stroller, 243–244; lightening of, 184; nutritional requirements of, 128–134, 135. *See also* nutrient(s); preparing breasts for, 105, 113–117; sleeping for, 166–168; visualizing life with, 160–161; what to have ready for, 180

Baby Blues (postpartum depression), 227, 233

baby hugs, 57

back: lying on, 8, 168, 197; muscles of, 45, 48, 50, 52, 69–72, 86, 87, 92, 93, 99, 240; strength training for, 69–72, 240; yoga stretch for, 99

back stretch, 99

backroom heat yoga, 83

basketball, 7

belly bra, 15, 36

belly support, 15

b-endorphin, xx

benefits of exercise, xv–xxvii, 18, 31, 82, 105–107, 228; baby and, xxi–xxii, 18; on delivery, xx–xxi, 18, 31; on emotional health, xix–xx; on labor, xx–xxi, 18, 31; in stress avoidance, xix, xxi, 82, 170

Berry, Amy, 82

biceps, 48–49, 63

biceps curl, 63

bicycle, 238

big day, 183–195; countdown to, 177–181; visualizing, 150–152

Bikram yoga, 83

Birth of a Mother: How the Motherhood Experience Changes You Forever (Stern and Brushweiler-Stern), 161

birth partner: acupressure and, 214, 216; birth plan and, 151; cesarean delivery and, 222; massage and, 210; positions for labor and delivery and, 198, 204, 205, 206; relaxation exercises and, 154–156; timing contractions and, 187

birth plan, 149–150, 178

birth weight: caffeine consumption and, 141; eating disorder and, 123; low weight gain and, 123; prenatal exercise and, xxvi–xxvii; stress and, 169

birthing ball, 200, 211–212

birthing bar, 206

birthing center: function of, 209–210; tour of, 151–152

blood flow: exercise and, xxv–xxvi; lying on back and, 197; yoga and, 87

BMI (Body Mass Index), 121, 122

body: changes in, during pregnancy, 8, 10–11; temperature of. *See* body temperature

Body Mass Index (BMI), 121, 122

body temperature: clothing and, 14–15; pregnancy and, xxvi, 14–15; regulation of, 139–140, 144; water and, 139–140

brachioradialis, 48–49

Braxton Hicks contractions, 184

bread, 136

breast(s). *See also* nipple(s): care of, 113–115; preparing for baby, 105, 113–117; support for, during exercise, 15–16

breast pumps, 116

breast shells, 116

breastfeeding. *See also* breast(s); nipple(s): contractions during, 230; education about, 116, 228; effects of exercise on, 242–243; first, 224

breathing: basics of, 157; beginning-stage techniques and, 189; deep, 172, 231; focal point and, 157; in labor, 153, 157–158; modified-pace, 158; pant-pant-blow, 158; patterns in, 157–158; relaxation and, 157; slow-pace, 158; in yoga, 83–84

Brushweiler-Stern, Nadia, 161

butterfly, 95

buttocks, strength training for, 52, 74, 76

C

caffeine, 129, 141, 167, 170

calcium, 130, 133, 137–138, 140, 141

calf muscles, 48, 94, 104

calf raises, 75

calming your mind, 172

calorie consumption, 123–124

carbohydrates, 134, 136–137; carbo-loading near delivery and, 142–143, 180; craving, 132; sources of, 136–137

carbo-loading, 142–143, 180

cardiovascular fitness, xiii, xiv, 19–39

career, motherhood and, 162–163

carpal tunnel syndrome (CTS), 61, 67

cat pose, 92

Centers for Disease Control and Prevention (CDC), xxiv, 129

cereal, 136

cervical effacement and dilation, 188–189, 190

cesarean section(s): birth plan and, 150; circumstances requiring, 221–222; epidurals and, 207; induction of labor and, 194; pre-natal exercises and, xxi; recovery from, 222, 230–231; side effects of, 222; spinal block and, 220; vaginal birth after (VBAC), 222; weight gain and, 119

chest muscles, 87, 97

cigarettes, 170

Clapp, James, III, xviii, xx, xxii, xxiv, xxvi, 5, 8, 43

cleansing breath, 157

clothing: for baby, 180; for exercising, 14–16; for yoga, 84

cognitive control, 156

cold compresses, 211

complex carbohydrates, 136

constipation, 133

consulting with health practitioner. *See also* keeping health practitioner informed: about birthing ball in delivery room, 211; about exercise, xiii, xxiv, 1, 3–4, 8, 240; about massage, 171; about need for episiotomy, 221; about positions for labor and delivery, 198; about when to head for hospital, 189; about yoga, 83; about your level of depression, 227

contraction(s): Braxton Hicks, 184; coping with, in first-stage labor, 198–205; duration of, 187; frequency of, 187; irregular and often painless, 184; pain from. *See* pain involved in labor and delivery; postpartum, 230; preterm, 13; timing chart and, 187, 188; timing of, 185, 186, 187–188; true labor or false labor and, 185, 186

cool-downs, 11, 12, 20, 22, 27, 31, 38, 42, 97, 241
CoolMax™, 15
crunch, incline, 60
C-section. *See* cesarean section
CTS (carpal tunnel syndrome), 61, 67
curls, 62–63, 240
cycling: clothing and, 14; form points for, 26; as non-weight-bearing cardiovascular exercise, 19, 26–30; safety and, 7–8, 17, 26–27; sample programs for, 27–30; tips for, 26

D

dairy products, 137–138
dangle, 204
deep breathing, 172, 231
dehydration, 13
delivery. *See also* labor: acupressure and, 213–216; benefits of exercise on, xx–xxi, 18, 31; birthing ball and, 211–212; birthing centers and, 209–210; cesarean. *See* cesarean section; day of. *See* big day; drug therapies and, xxi, 217, 218–221. *See also* drugs; epidural block; first hour after, 190; forceps use in, 207, 221; getting set for, 147–158; hydrotherapy and, 212; medical interventions in, 217–222. *See also* individual interventions; music and, 216; natural supports and, 207–216; pain involved in. *See* pain involved in labor and delivery; of placenta, 188, 190, 191; positions for, 197–206, 211; premature, xviii; recovery after. *See* recovery; vacuum use in, 207, 221

deltoids, 48–49
Demerol, 218–219
depression: postpartum (Baby Blues), 227, 233; during pregnancy, xix–xx, 166
diabetes: gestational, xviii, 119; type I, 2
diarrhea, 133, 184
diastasis recti, 56–57
diet. *See* eating
dilation of cervix, 188–189, 190
doctor. *See* health practitioner
doula, 209
downhill skiing, 7
downward dog, 91
dress. *See* clothing
Dri-FIT™, 15
drinking: avoidance of alcohol and, 129, 141, 142, 167, 170, 179; in labor, 193; need for hydration during pregnancy and, 13–14, 133–134, 139–140, 144, 193
drugs: epidural and. *See* epidural block; narcotics and, 218–219; nitrous oxide and, 219; pain medication and, 218–219, 226, 230; prenatal exercises and, xxi; pudendal block and, 219–220; spinal block and, 220

E

eating. *See also* food(s): after first breastfeeding, 224; calorie consumption and, 123–124; control and, 120–128. *See also* weight management; eating disorder and, 123; healthier choices in, 126–128; in labor, 143, 193; meal planning and, 144–145; nutritional requirements and, 128–134, 135. *See also* nutrient(s);

serving size and, 123–124; for two, 119–145
eating disorder, 123
education: breastfeeding, 116, 228. *See also* breast(s); nipple(s); parenting classes and, 158–159, 178; prenatal classes and, 147–149, 178
effacement of cervix, 188–189
eggs, 129, 137
Elevator Kegel exercise, 109–110
emotional health, benefits of exercise on, xix–xx
endurance, 19, 44
epidural block, xi, 150, 190; description of, 218; disadvantages of, 207–208; side effects of, 207–208, 218
episiotomy, 50, 110–111, 219, 220–221, 235
Equilibrium Fitness, 82
exercise: aerobic. *See* aerobic exercises; benefits of. *See* benefits of exercise; miscarriage and, xxiv–xxv, 4; postpartum. *See* postpartum exercise(s); during pregnancy. *See* prenatal exercise(s); prenatal. *See* prenatal exercise(s); preterm labor and, xxiv–xxv; relaxation, 154–156, 172–173
exercise band, 84
Exercising Through Your Pregnancy (Clapp), xviii
exhaustion, 132
external electronic monitoring, 194

F
Family Medicine Magazine, 148
fatigue, 132, 169, 235
fats, 114, 134, 138–139
feet, putting up, 168–169

Fetal Alcohol Syndrome, 142
fetal monitoring, 188, 190, 193–194
fish, 138
Fit Pregnancy Magazine, 21
fitness. *See also* exercise: cardiovascular, xiii, xiv, 19–39; current, assessing, 4–5; in pregnancy, basics of, 1–18
flapping fish pose, 96
flat ab exercises, 237, 238, 239
flexibility training, xiii, xvi, xvii, xviii, 12–13, 81. *See also* yoga
focal point, 157
folate (vitamin B9), 129, 135, 141
folic acid, 129, 140
food(s). *See also* eating; nutrient(s): to avoid, 141–142; food guidelines and, 124–125, 129; meal planning and, 144–145; pregnancy and, 13, 119–145; prenatal exercises and, 13
Food and Drug Administration, 138
forceps, 207, 221
forward bend, 87
free weights, 42, 49
fruits, 136–137

G
gastrocnemius, 75
Gatorade™, 140, 143, 193
gestational diabetes, xviii, 119
"giggle gas," 219
glycogen, 41–42, 134, 142, 143, 228
guided relaxation, 154–155
gymnastics, 7

H
hamstrings, 48, 49, 52, 76, 87, 94, 103
hand exercises, 67–68
hands and knees position during labor, 201

health practitioner: consulting with. *See* consulting with health practitioner; going over birth plan with, 150, 178; keeping informed. *See* keeping health practitioner informed
heart rate, exercise intensity and, xxii–xxiv
heartburn, 133, 166, 167
hemorrhoids, 106, 133
hip extensions, 76
hips: strength training for, 74, 76; yoga stretch for, 100
hockey, ice, 7
Hoffman Technique, 116
horseback riding, 7
hospital, tour of, 151–152. *See also* birthing center
hospital bag, packing, 181
hot compresses, 211
hydrotherapy, 212
hypnosis, 152–153

I
ice hockey, 7
incline crunch, 60
indigestion, 133
induction of labor, 194–195
intermittent external monitoring, 193–194
internal electronic monitoring, 194
intravenous oxytocin, 190
intravenous pitocin, 195
inverted nipples, 114; checking for, 113, 115–116, 178; correction methods and, 116
iron, 133, 135, 138, 140, 141
iron deficiency (anemia), 2, 132, 137, 140

J
jogging stroller, 243–244
Jones, Shelle, 69
Journal of Women's Health, xix
Joy, Elizabeth, xix, 27, 36, 37, 56

K
Katz, Jane, 31–32
keeping health practitioner informed. *See also* consulting with health practitioner: about feeling need to vomit as baby's head presses on cervix, 184–185; about labor symptoms, 185, 186; about postpartum warning signs, 225; about signs of approaching labor, 184
Kegel, Arnold, 107
Kegel exercises, xvi, xvii–xviii, 107–110; benefits of, 105–107; pelvic bulging and, 109–110, 179; during postpartum period, 106, 107, 228, 235, 240; tips for, 108
KY Jelly™, 112

L
La Leche League, 113–114, 116, 117, 160
labor. *See also* delivery: acupressure and, 213–216; approaching, signs of, 179, 183–185; benefits of exercise on, xx–xxi, 18, 31; birthing ball and, 211–212; birthing centers and, 209–210; breathing in, 153, 157–158; coping at home and, 185–186; doula and, 209; drinking in, 193; drug therapies and, xxi,

217, 218–221. *See also* drugs; epidural block; eating in, 143, 193; getting set for, 147–158; hot and cold compresses and, 211; hydrotherapy and, 212; induction of, 194–195; keeping hydrated during, 144, 193; length of, 191; massage during, 210; medical interventions in, 217–222. *See also* individual interventions; midwife and, 208–209, 210; music and, 216; pain involved in. *See* pain involved in labor and delivery; positions for, 197–206, 211; preterm. *See* preterm labor; signs of, 179, 183–185; stages of. *See* labor, stage(s) of; T.E.N.S. (Transcutaneous Electrical Nerve Stimulation) and, 213; three stages of. *See* stage(s) of labor; true or false?, 185, 186
labor, stage(s) of: first, 188–189, 198–205; second, 188, 190, 206; third, 188, 190
Lansinoh™, 114, 226
lateral raises, 65
latissimus, 45, 48, 71
leg lifts, 77
leg slides, 228–229
leg stretch, 94
legs: muscles of, 48, 73–77, 89, 92, 94; strength training for, 73–77; strengthening with yoga, 89
lightening, 184
lochia, 230
loss of mucus plug, 179, 184
lower back muscles, 45, 48, 50, 52, 93

lumbar lordosis, 69
lunges, 74; walking, 43
lying on back, 8, 168, 197

M

Madonna, 82, 244
manual perineum stretching, xvi, xvii, 105, 110–112
massage, 170–171, 174; during labor, 210; perineal, xvi, xvii, 105, 110–112, 178
maternal fever, 207
maternity bra, 16, 114
meat, 129, 137, 138
medical professional. *See* health practitioner
Melbourne, University of, xx
Melpomene Institute, xxiv, 36, 235
membranes: rupturing, 195; stripping, 195
mercury, 138
Michigan, University of, xix
mid-back muscles, 93
midwife, 208–209, 210. *See also* health practitioner
mind, calming, 172
minerals, 140–141
miscarriage, xxiv–xxv, 4
Misconceptions: Truth, Lies, and the Unexpected on the Journey to Motherhood (Wolf), 191
modified ab workout, 236
modified-pace breathing, 158
"mommy tendonitis," 61
"morning" sickness, 129, 130–131, 132, 166
motherhood: career and, 162–163; getting set for, 158–163; nesting instinct and, 174–175, 185;

motherhood: *continued*
    setting aside control and, 161–162; support networks and, 159–160
Mothers in Motion™, 15
motivation tips, 17
mucus plug, loss of, 179, 184
muscle(s), 44–49; abdominal, 45, 50, 52, 56–60, 92, 228, 235–239; arm, 48–49, 61–68, 86, 87, 92, 240; back, 45, 48, 50, 52, 69–72, 86, 87, 92, 93, 99, 240; calf, 48, 94, 104; chest, 87, 97; hamstring, 48, 49, 52, 76, 87, 94, 103; illustrated, 46–47; leg, 48, 73–77, 89, 92, 94; neck, 85, 99, 229; pelvic floor. *See* pelvic floor muscles; shoulder, 69–72, 85, 86, 92, 229, 240; strengthening. *See* strength training
music, 216

N

nap, 167, 168, 179, 181, 186, 224. *See also* rest; sleep
narcotics, 218–219
National Institutes of Health, 130
National Sleep Foundation (NSF), 165, 166–167
nausea, 129, 130–131, 132, 166, 184–185, 213
neck muscles, 85, 99, 229
nesting instinct, 174–175, 185
nipple(s). *See also* breast(s): care of, 113–115; inverted. *See* inverted nipples; preparing for baby, 113–117; soreness of, from breastfeeding, 225–226; stimulation of, to induce labor, 195
nipple shields, 116
nitrous oxide, 219

NSF (National Sleep Foundation), 165, 166–167
nursery accessories, 180
nursing bra, 114, 115, 179
nutrient(s), 128–134. *See also* individual nutrients; critical, listed, 135; nausea and, 130–131; tips regarding, 144

O

obliques, 45, 56, 58
Obstetrics and Gynecology, 111, 119
open spinal twist, 93
oxygen, exercise and, xxv–xxvi, 18
oxytocin, 190, 195

P

packing hospital bag, 181
Padron, Sasha, 148
pain involved in labor and delivery: epidural and. *See* epidural block; narcotics and, 218–219; natural supports to lessen, 208–216; truth about, 191–192
pain medication, 218–219, 226, 230
pant-pant-blow breathing, 158
parenting classes, 158–159, 178
Parker, Sarah Jessica, 244
pasta, 136
pelvic bulging, 109–110, 179
pelvic circles, 88
pelvic floor muscles, 45, 50; conditioning of, benefits of, 105–107, 228. *See also* Kegel exercises; finding, 107–108
pelvic rock, 52–55, 228
pelvic tilts, 52–55, 228
perineal massage, xvi, xvii, 105, 110–112, 178
perineal tearing, xvi, 106, 110, 111, 220, 221

perineum stretching, xvi, xvii, 105, 110–112
physician. *See* health practitioner
pitocin, 195
placenta: blood flow to, 197; delivery of, 188, 190, 191; tearing away from uterine wall (placenta abruption), 222; vagina blocked by (placenta previa), 221–222
placenta abruption, 222
placenta previa, 221–222
plow, 241–242
postpartum depression (Baby Blues), 227, 233
postpartum exercise(s): aerobic, 240–241; after cesarean delivery, 231; after vaginal birth, 106, 107, 228–229; consulting with health practitioner about, 240; contraindications to, 234; cool-downs and, 241; effects of, on breastfeeding, 242–243; getting back in the game and, 233–244; in-bed, 106, 107, 228–229; stretching and, 229, 241; warm-ups and, 241; when to start, 234–235; yoga and, 204–242
postpartum warning signs, 225
posture: poor, characteristics of, 78; sitting, 80; for sleep, 96, 168; standing, 79; strength training for, 78–80; for walking, 21
potassium, 133, 135, 136, 137, 140, 143
preeclampsia, xviii, 2, 119, 221
pregnancy: body changes during, 8, 10–11; depression in, xix–xx, 166; exercise after. *See* postpartum exercise(s); exercise during. *See* prenatal exercise(s); fitness and. *See* fitness; food and, 13, 119–145.

See also eating; food(s); hydration and, 13–14, 133–134, 139–140, 144, 193
pregnancy belt, 15
prelabor, 184
premature delivery, xviii
prenatal classes, 147–149, 178
prenatal exercise(s). *See also* strength training: aerobic, 19–39. *See also* cycling; running; swimming; walking; beginners and, 8; benefits of, xv–xxvii, 18, 31; blood flow and, xxv–xxvi; body temperature and, xxvi, 14, 30; cardiovascular, 19–39. *See also* cycling; running; swimming; walking; clothing for, 14–16; commitment to, 17–18; components of, xiii; consulting with health practitioner about, xiii, xxiv, 1, 3–4, 8; contraindications to, 1–3; cool-downs and, 11, 12, 20, 22, 27, 31, 38, 42, 97; in first-stage labor, 198–205; food and, 13; frequency of, 5; hydration and, 13–14; intensity of, xxii–xxiv, 6–7; limitations on, xxiii; locations for, 16–17; motivation and, 17; oxygen and, xxv–xxvi, 18; relaxation, 154–156, 172–173; safety and, xxii–xxvii, 5–7, 8, 9, 16–17; in second-stage labor, 206; session duration and, 5; stretching and, 12–13, 97–104. *See also* yoga; types of, 7–8. *See also* individual sports and types of exercise; warm-ups and, 11–12, 20, 22, 27, 31, 38, 42, 97; when to stop, 7; yoga and, 81–104. *See also* yoga
prenatal nausea, 129, 130–131, 132, 166, 213
prenatal yoga. *See* yoga

prenatal yoga pose sequence, 85–96
the press-and-reach, 237
preterm contractions, 13
preterm labor: dehydration and, 13; exercise and, xxiv–xxv; nipples and, 114; stress and, 169
progesterone, 166
prostaglandin, 195
protein, 114, 134, 135, 137, 181
pudenal block, 219–220

Q
quadriceps, 48, 50, 101, 102

R
racket sports, 7
Rating of Perceived Exertion Scale (RPE), 6, 20, 22, 27, 44
Recommended Pregnancy Weight Gain charts, 121–123
recovery, 223–232; first few hours after delivery and, 224; first few days after delivery and, 226, 228; first three weeks after delivery and, 229–230; body image during, 231–232; from cesarean delivery, 222, 230–231; postpartum warning signs and, 225; from vaginal birth, 224–230
rectus abdominis, 45, 56, 57; separated, 236
rectus muscle separation test, 56–57
reflexology, 171
relaxation: breathing and, 157; exercises for, 154–156, 172–173; guided, 154–155; promotion of, with yoga, 85, 86, 93, 94; systemic, 154–155
relaxin, 12, 83
resistance training. *See* strength training

rest. *See also* sleep: getting needed, 167–168, 224, 226, 227, 229–230; power of, 165–175; putting feet up and, 168–169
reverse curl, 62
rhomboids, 48
rice, 136
RPE (Rating of Perceived Exertion Scale), 6, 20, 22, 27, 44
rubber-band row, 71, 240
running, 73; with baby in jogging stroller, 243–244; clothing and, 14; form tips for, 37; safety and, 7–8, 16–17; sample program for, 38–39; tips for, 37; as weight-bearing cardiovascular exercise, 19, 36–39
rupturing membranes, 195

S
salt, 142, 167
scuba diving, 7
Sea Bands™, 131, 213
seafood, 138
self-hypnosis, 153
semi-sitting position during labor, 202, 206
serving size, 123–124
Sharpe, Mary, 229
shins, yoga stretch for, 100
shoulder rolls, 86, 229
shoulder shrugs, 72
shoulder-blade squeeze, 70, 240
shoulders: muscles of, 69–72, 85, 86, 92, 229, 240; strength training for, 69–72, 240
side reaches, 58
side-lying position during labor, 203, 206
simple carbohydrates, 136
sitting: during labor, 200; posture for, 80; semi-, during labor, 202, 206

skiing, downhill, 7
sleep. *See also* rest: getting needed, 167–168, 224, 226, 227, 229–230; nap and, 167, 168, 179, 181, 186, 224; posture for, 96, 168; tips for, 167; for two, 166–168; when baby sleeps, 226, 227
slow-dancing, 205
slow-pace breathing, 158
soccer, 7
soleus, 75
spinal block, 220
spinal erectors, 45, 48
spinal rolls, 90
spinal twist, open, 93
sports bra, 16
squatting: as best position for labor and delivery, 206, 211; learning, 49–50; strength training and, 49–51; tips for, 50
Stadol, 218–219
standing: during labor, 199; posture for, 79; yoga and, 7, 83
Stern, Daniel N., 160–161
strength training, xiii, 41–80; abdominal work in, 56–60; for arms, 61–68, 240; for back and shoulders, 69–72, 240; basics of, 42–49; beginning, 44; cool-downs and, 42, 97; equipment for, 42, 49; frequency of, 42; for legs, 73–77; muscles and. *See* muscle(s); pelvic rock and, 52–55; postpartum, 240; for shoulders and back, 69–72, 240; squatting and, 49–51. *See also* squatting; tips for, 43; warm-ups and, 42, 97
stress: avoiding, 148, 165, 169–174; benefits of exercise and, xix, xxi, 82, 170

stretching. *See also* yoga: perineum, xvi, xvii, 105, 110–112; postpartum, 229, 241; prenatal, 12–13, 97–104
stripping membranes, 195
sugar, 142, 167
supine hypotensive syndrome, 8
swimming: body temperature and, 14; as non-weight-bearing cardiovascular exercise, 19, 30–35; safety and, 7–8; sample programs for, 32–35; tips for, 32
swollen ankles, 134, 167
systemic relaxation, 154–155

T

talk test, 6
temperature, body. *See* body temperature
T.E.N.S. (Transcutaneous Electrical Nerve Stimulation), 213
thighs: strength training for, 74, 77; strengthening with yoga, 90
thoracic kyphosis, 69
toe-flexing exercises, 231
tofu, 138
toiletries for baby, 180
topical prostaglandin, 195
training: defined, xii–xiii; resistance. *See* strength training; strength. *See* strength training
Transcutaneous Electrical Nerve Stimulation (T.E.N.S.), 213
transverse abdominis, 45, 57
trapezius, 48
triceps, 48–49, 66, 98
triceps extensions, 66
tuna, 138
type I diabetes, 2

U

United States Department of Agriculture (USDA), Food Guide Pyramid of, 124–125
University of Melbourne, xx
University of Michigan, xix
University of Utah, xix
upper back muscles, 48, 86
upper body, yoga stretch for, 98
USDA (United States Department of Agriculture), Food Guide Pyramid of, 124–125
Utah, University of, xix

V

vacuum, 207, 221
vagina: after birth, 230; blocked by placenta (placenta previa), 221–222; preparing, 105–112
vaginal birth after cesarean (VBAC), 222
vaginal tearing, 50, 106, 110–111, 220, 221
Valsalva maneuver, 43
VBAC (vaginal birth after cesarean), 222
vegetables, 136–137
visualization: of big day, 150–152; of life with baby, 160–161
vitamin(s), 140–141; A, 140; B9 (folate), 129, 135, 141

W

waist twists, 89
walking, 73; with baby in jogging stroller, 243–244; beginners and, 8; cooling down and, 12; in labor, 198–199; posture tips for, 21; safety and, 7–8; sample programs for, 22–25; tips for, 21; as weight-bearing cardiovascular exercise, 19, 20–25
walking lunges, 43
warm-ups, 11–12, 20, 22, 27, 31, 38, 42, 97, 241
water: body temperature and, 139–140; giving birth in, 212; need for, during pregnancy, 13–14, 133–134, 139–140, 144, 193
Water Fitness Through Your Pregnancy (Katz), 31
Wave Kegel exercise, 109, 110
weight: excess, gaining, xv, xviii, 8, 18, 119; ideal, 122; low, 123; management of. *See* weight management; postpartum loss of, 231–232; starting, 120–121, 123
weight management: Body Mass Index (BMI) and, 121, 122; exercise and, xv, xviii–xix, 8, 18; importance of, 120; Recommended Pregnancy Weight Gain charts and, 121–123; starting point and, 120–121, 123
weights, free, 42, 49
Wolf, Naomi, 191
wrist curl, 62, 240

Y

yoga, xvi, xvii, xviii, 81–104; backroom heat, 83; basic stretches in, 97–104; beginning, 83; benefits of, 82; Bikram, 83; breathing and, 83–84; consulting with health practitioner about, 83; coping with stress and, 82, 170; do's and don'ts in, 83; equipment for, 84; postpartum, 204–242; prenatal pose sequence in, 85–96; standing and, 7, 83
yoga mat, 84
yoga pose sequence, 85–96
Yoga Space, 148
yoga strap, 84